MAKEUP
marie claire

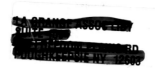

MAKEUP

marie claire

HEARST BOOKS

A division of Sterling Publishing Co., Inc.

New York / London
www.sterlingpublishing.com

Contents

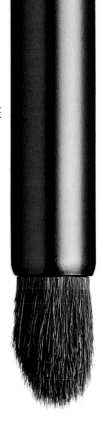

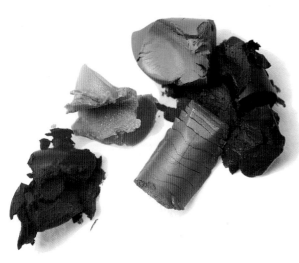

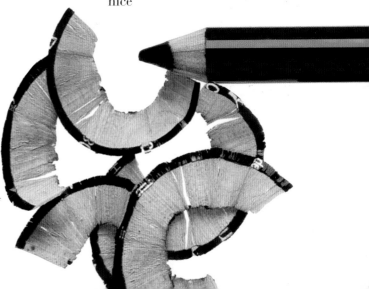

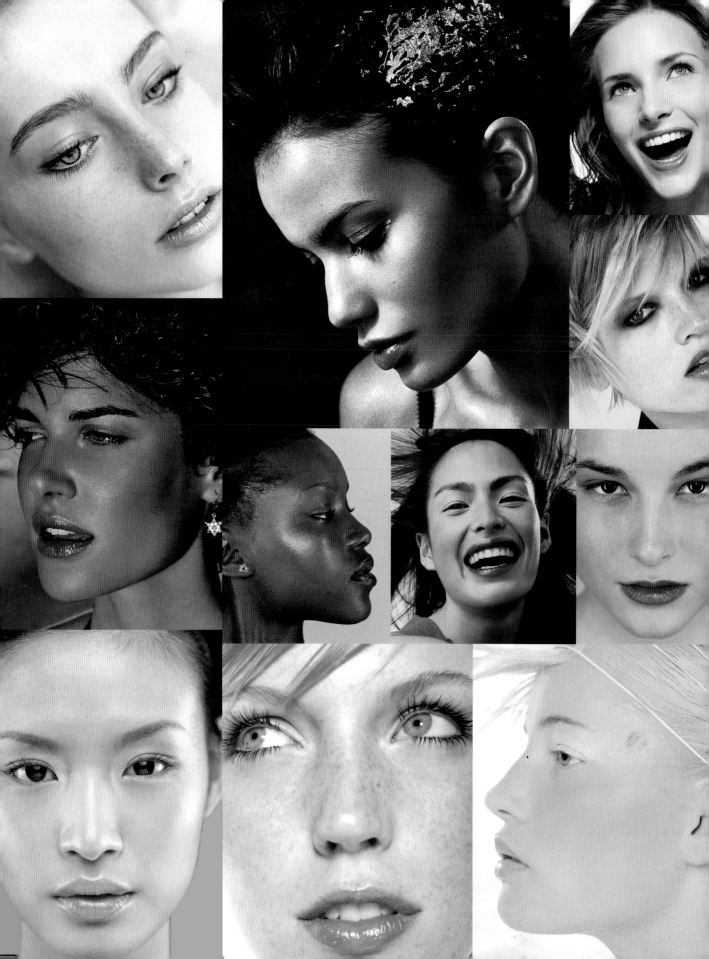

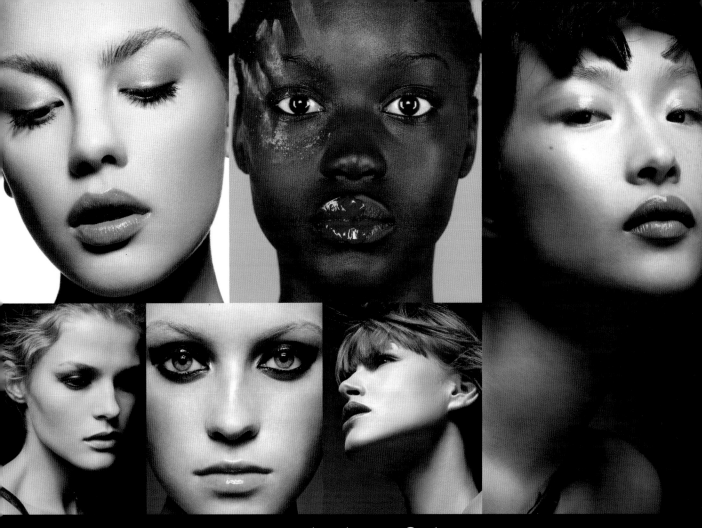

A world of beauty . . .

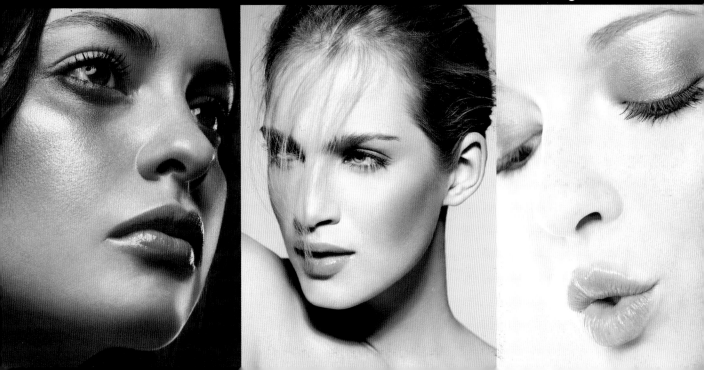

1

THE SKIN YOU'RE IN

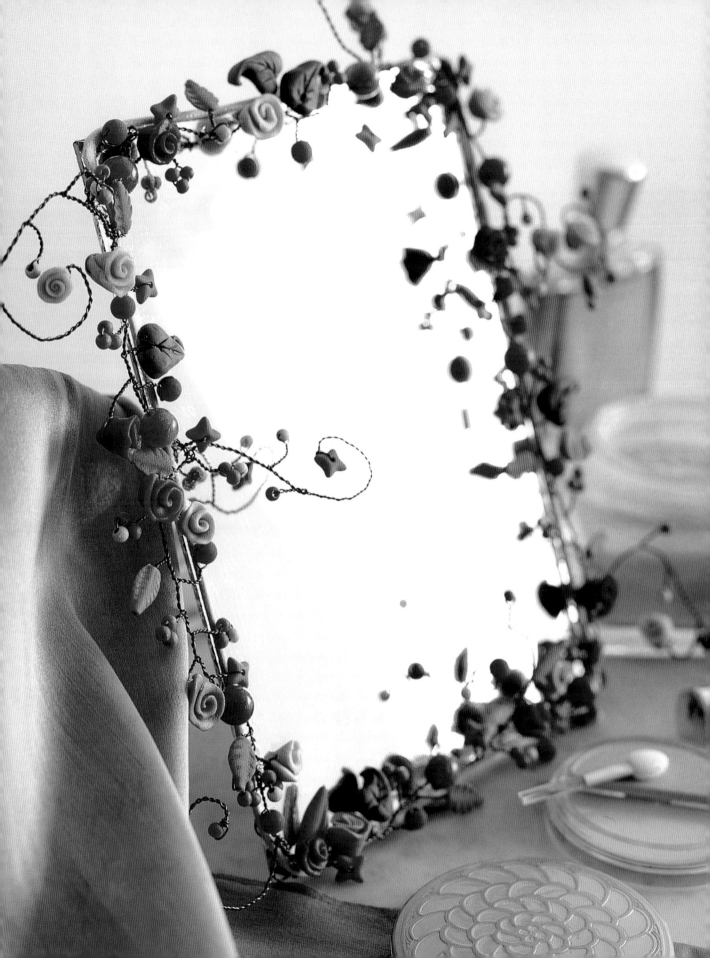

Made-for-you hues

Find the makeup palette that suits your skin tone.

FAIR Accentuate milky skin with pearly white, translucent beige, and rosy pink tones. If your skin is on the pinkish side, look for rosy foundation and copper bronzing powder; if it's more yellowish opt for golden hues.

MEDIUM-GOLDEN Gold and copper shades bring out the natural beauty of your skin tone.

MEDIUM-DARK Women with this type of coloring should opt for orange or rosy beige tones to create contrast.

BROWN TO BLACK Small bursts of color enliven and give contour and vitality to your skin.

It's genetic: Melanin, a natural pigment, is the primary determinant of human skin color. There are 10 basic tones used to classify white skin but over 80 for black skin. The color depends on how much light is reflected or absorbed by these tones. Most light is reflected off "white" skin, making it appear lighter. On the other hand, the more melanin present, the more light the skin will absorb, producing an increasingly dark color.

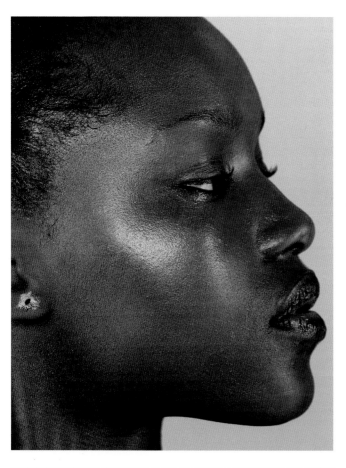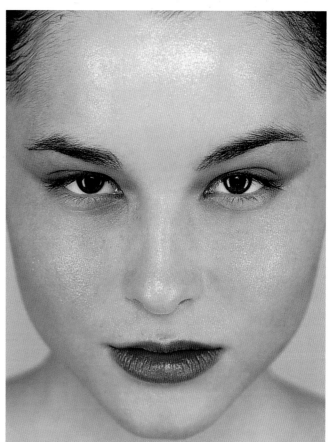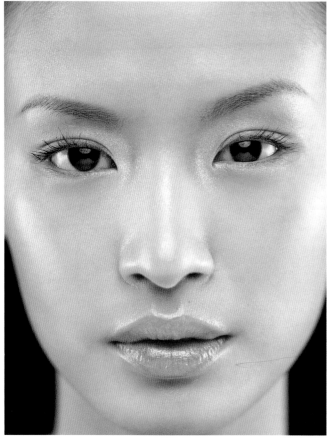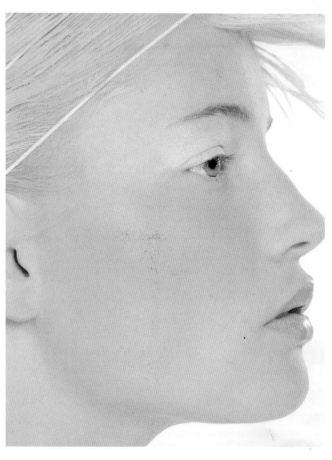

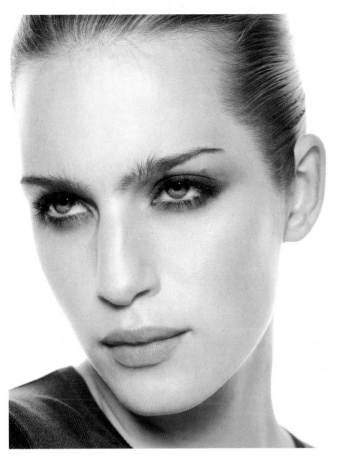
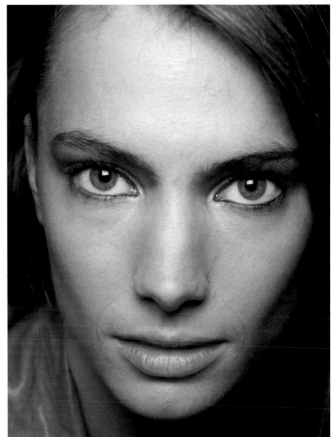
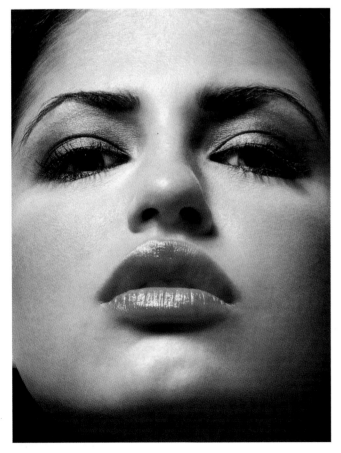
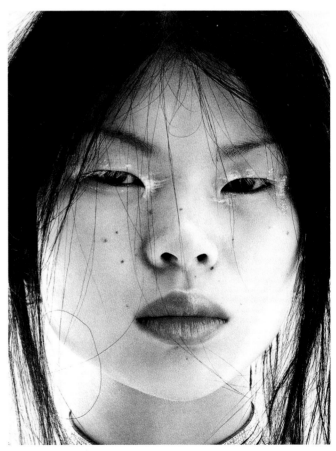

Know your facial structure

In modern society beauty is not based on a particular face shape.
Vive la différence! The one simple rule: make the best of what you have.

OVAL This is the perfect face of ages past: eyes separated by an eye's length, a forehead wider than the lower face, and eyebrows that arch just above the middle of your eyes. Use makeup to help bring out your personality by highlighting either your eyes or your lips.

RECTANGULAR Horizontal lines will help give your face more width and vivacity. Shorter and less-arched eyebrows also help. Blush should always go below your cheekbones.

TRIANGULAR Enhance a wide forehead and a small, narrow chin by accenting your cheekbones and filling out your eyebrows.

SQUARE Sweeping your brush upward toward your temples can minimize a harsh jaw line and soften the lines of your face. Generous eyebrow shaping toward the outer edges of your eyes will also help.

ROUND It's all about creating an illusion of length—fuller cheeks tend to appear more slender if you apply makeup in upward strokes. Keep your eyebrows on the thick side and as tapered outward as possible.

ANGULAR Drawing your eyebrows out toward your temples will soften geometric facial features.

ADVICE FROM A PROFESSIONAL MAKEUP ARTIST (Stila)
All faces are different, and, thankfully, there are no general rules that everyone must follow. If you close your eyes and explore the unique curves and contours of your own face, you will intuitively know what to accent.

Your eye color

The mirror of your emotions, a subtle palette that expresses the many nuances of your personality, a decisive weapon that you can magnify through countless combinations of colors and styles.

BLUE A marvelous optical illusion graces you with the most celebrated of eye colors. Blue eyes exist because low quantities of melanin and the action of chromosome 15 make the iris reflect light much as a lake would. Take advantage of this by favoring warmer tones like navy, smoky gray, chocolate, apricot, or copper.

GREEN Chromosome 19 affords you this pretty and rare eye color. From mauve to plum, all red-based hues will add fire to your gaze. Opposites attract, as they say...

GRAY This shade is a beautiful blank canvas that can reflect your mood. Want your eyes to appear blue? Gray or coppery red will do the trick. Feeling green? Dress in lavender or aquamarine.

HAZEL Warm, sandy tones ranging from beige to brown and very dark eyelashes will complement these brilliant peepers, as will all plum, purple, and green-bronze tones.

BLACK The rainbow's spectrum offers itself to you, but beware of too-light or pearly tones that can unflatteringly discolor the whites of your eyes. Midnight blue, dark gray, brown, or buff tones will accentuate the mystery of dark eyes.

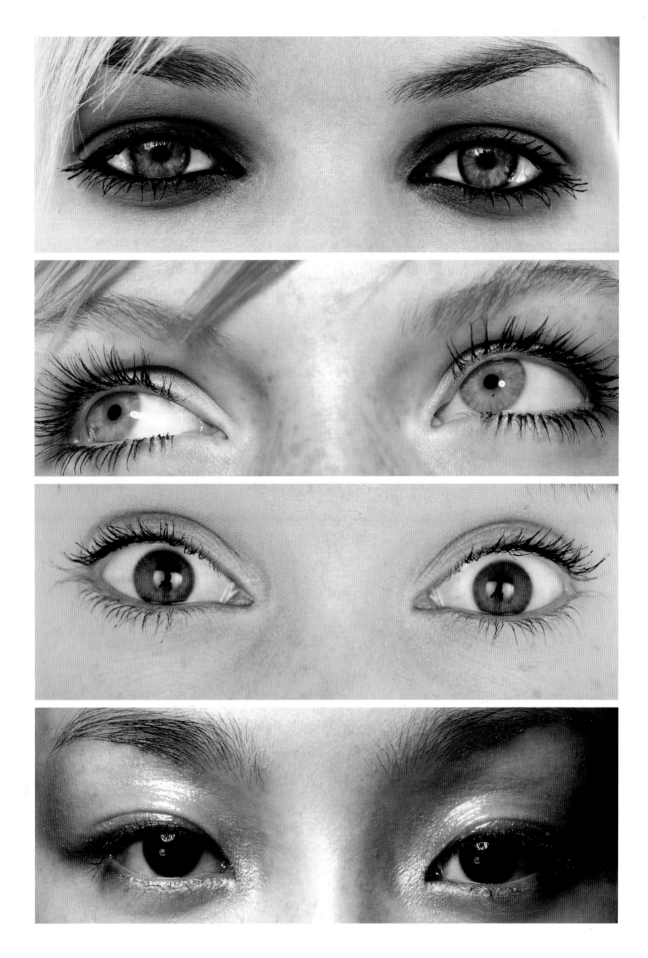

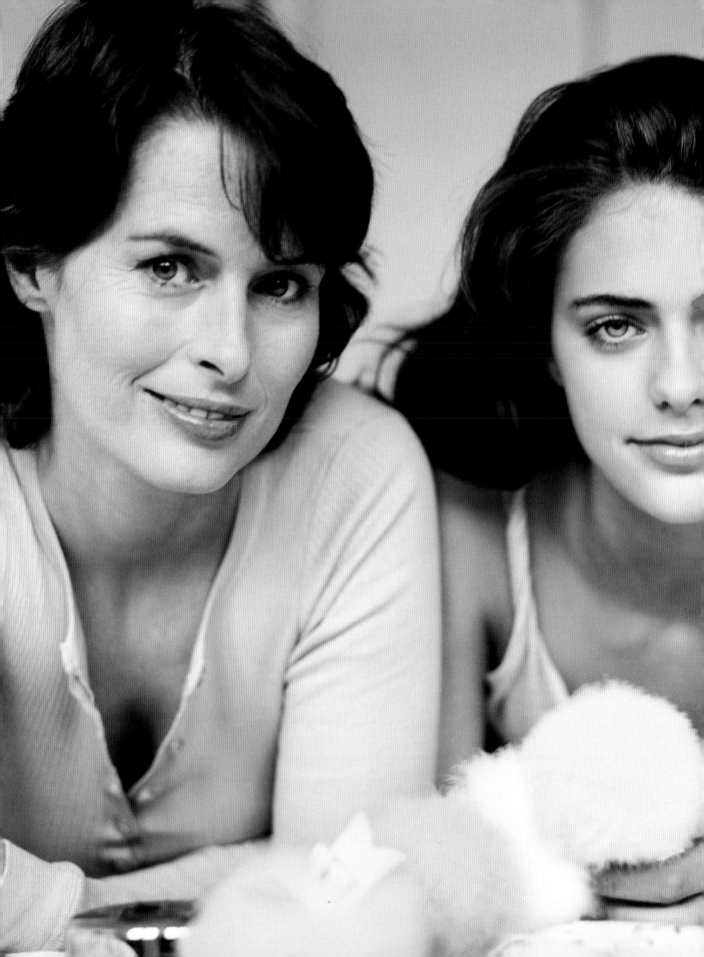

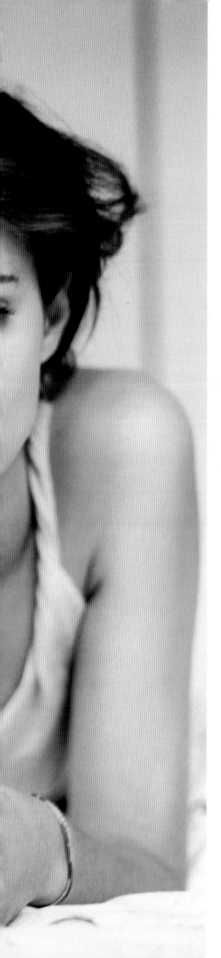

Gorgeous at every age!

Growing old gracefully and effortlessly, rekindling your beauty at any age: today's cosmetic industry has integrated all this and more into products which enhance your natural look. Here is a radiant example of mother-daughter mirror images…

A blissful beauty session at the spa shows that the generation gap is indeed closing. An increasing awareness of the importance of lifelong health and dietary consciousness is changing the way we age. And the ever-improving science of cosmetics is dedicated to lasting good looks.

THE NEW BREAKDOWN: YOUR BEAUTY REGIME

15-20 years old Know what you've got and take advantage of it.

30 years old You know what you want and what textures and formulas you prefer.

40 years old You're living *la dolce vita*: refine a few things and rediscover yourself.

50 years old and beyond You want it all and like being surprised.

THE UNDER-20 DEPARTMENT

It's useless to swipe mom's makeup and beauty products: now is the time to favor freshness and simplicity. At this age your assets are immense. Don't hide them under a layer of makeup.

▶

Complexion

• Use tinted moisturizer for a well-blended, even finish that won't clog your pores.

• Luminizing powder covers up minor imperfections.

• Use cheek stain that doubles as lip stain.

Eyes

• Soft-tipped pencils are undeniably the best tool at your age. They won't tug on your eyelids (which causes wrinkling later), and they come in a variety of vivid colors.

• Don't play with your eyebrows—changing their natural shape now could lead to long-term regrets.

Lips

• No need for artificial "plumping": gloss or shine are preferable to an overdone lipstick. A beige or pink hydrating lip balm combines treatment and glam results.

IN YOUR 30s AND 40s—WAYS TO FRESHEN YOUR LOOK

The secret Use small bursts of effective highlighting. Makeup can help you brighten these strategic spots:

• Nasolabial folds—the creases that run from your nose to the corners of your mouth
• "Lion" wrinkles—between the eyebrows
• Inner corners of your eyes
• Eyelid creases
• Contours of your mouth

AS YOU GET OLDER, GO EASY!

Complexion

Foundation should be used with caution: as the face grows older, it needs more light but certainly not heavy layers of makeup. New cosmetic formulas that let your skin breathe and

Powder puff pointers

Mastering powder application is an art: as long as you apply it with the lightness of a feather, the velvety or matte look it affords will greatly enhance your skin. Restricting its application to the middle of the face will guarantee a smooth finish and avoid creating a frozen expression.

▶

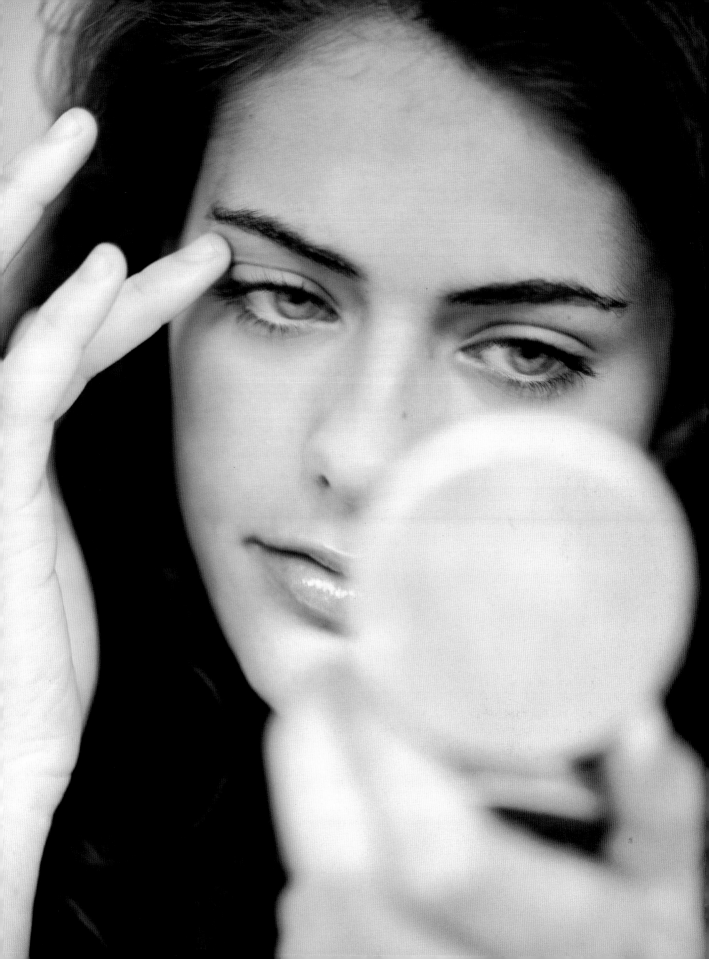

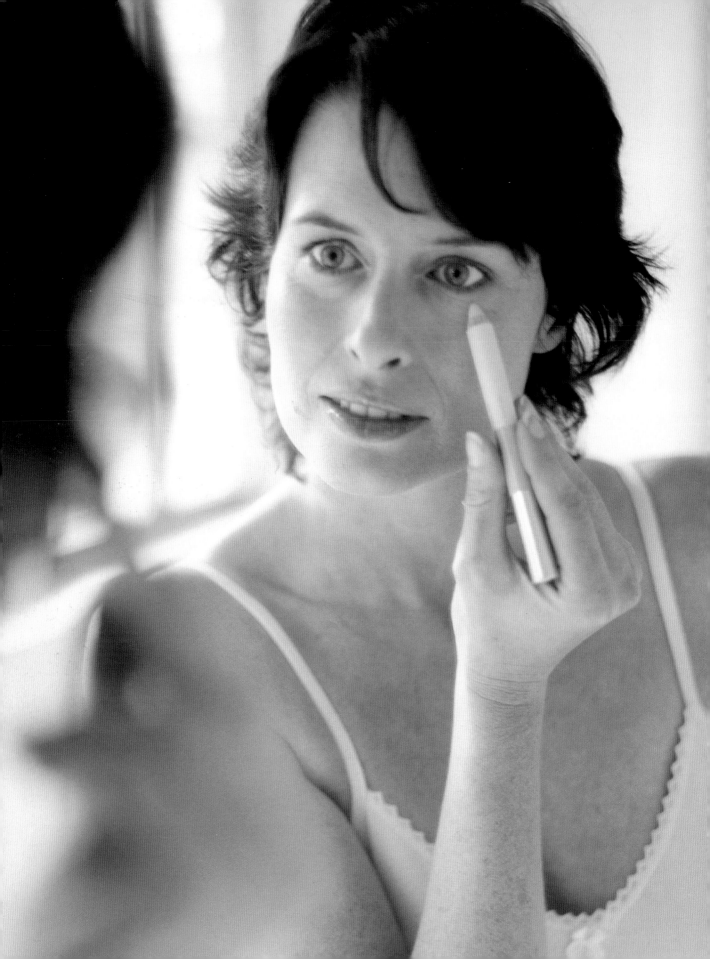

add radiance will give you a professional look without appearing too heavy. A mix of concealer and foundation, always a half-tone lighter than your skin, will sweep away shadows from:

- Inner corners of your eyes
- Nasolabial folds
- Contours of the mouth
- Below the lower lip

A concealer stick used sparingly will cover minor flaws, but be careful to only spot where necessary—aim for natural coverage.

Hint: Nothing is better than ice cubes to liven up your complexion and stimulate your lymphatic system. Always use ice wrapped in a towel to avoid burning your skin.

Eyes

- Beware of overdoing your eyeshadow: powder can build up in the small expressive wrinkles around the eyes, making them much more visible than without any makeup.
- Dusky, matte shadows bring out the sparkle in your eyes.
- Accentuate your eyebrows: fill them in toward your temples.
- Drawing a thin line along the inner rims of your eyes with an off-white kohl pencil will make your eyes look bigger and prevent yellowish reflections on the cornea.
- Brown or gray mascara is less aggressive and just as dramatic as black.

Lips

- Use a moisturizing lip balm and a lip contour treatment. Leave it on as long as possible to hydrate lips and banish small wrinkles.
- Try a lip-shaping pencil. Opt for a fat tip and follow the outer edge of your lips, stopping before the corners to avoid caking.
- Pearly pink eyeshadow can be used on your lips in combination with a red semi-gloss.

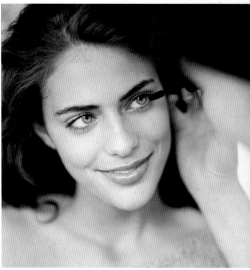

A single coat of mascara and you're good to go!

The future of beauty

Here's to science! Biologist Gérard Redziniak from Pacific Creation gave us an overview of what's looming on the horizon.

TOMORROW'S MIRROR just might be a computer with a built-in camera that will manage your colors according to your mood or a particular celebrity look that you want to create on a given day. **LASER TECHNOLOGY** will help you pick the best mascara or identify and banish problem wrinkles before they develop. Biology and cosmetic science will unite to create clarifiers and concealers that will afford you flawless skin. **ABSOLUTE MOISTURIZERS** and **SECOND-SKIN FORMULAS** will be commonplace, as will infinitely natural-looking masks. Light-diffusing, soft-focus complexion enhancers will cause light to bounce off the skin at the angle it shines on you. **CLEAR LIQUID CRYSTALS,** like those in LCD screens, will enhance this "radiance" and reflect **DAZZLINGLY MAGNIFICENT COLORS** using Polaroid techniques in which invisible particles protect your skin while giving off a suntanned glow… We'll be chameleons with makeup that adapts to our surroundings and circumstances. "Smart" foundations will identify problem areas and correct them before they become visible. An **UTTERLY CLEAR LIPSTICK,** whose active ingredients will morph from the **SHEEREST GLOSS TO THE DEEPEST RED,** will present an infinite range of possibilities in respect to available light…instantly generating a **PROTECTIVE POLYMER PLUMPING FILM** directly on the lips. You decide between simple and natural or the most dramatic looks imaginable. Chemistry will also help by creating freeze-drying techniques that yield extremely pure powders, or molecular encapsulation that produces sun screens and dyes that never come into direct contact with the skin because they are locked in miniscule glass pearls: a limitless color palette at your fingertips, not possible today because of toxicity concerns. Polymers and other **MICROSCOPIC PARTICLES, SUCH AS MINI LIGHT TUBES OR DIODES THAT ILLUMINATE YOUR SKIN FOR AN EVENING,** will highlight specific features. Finally, we'll be able to create the effect of diamonds without even piercing our ears…

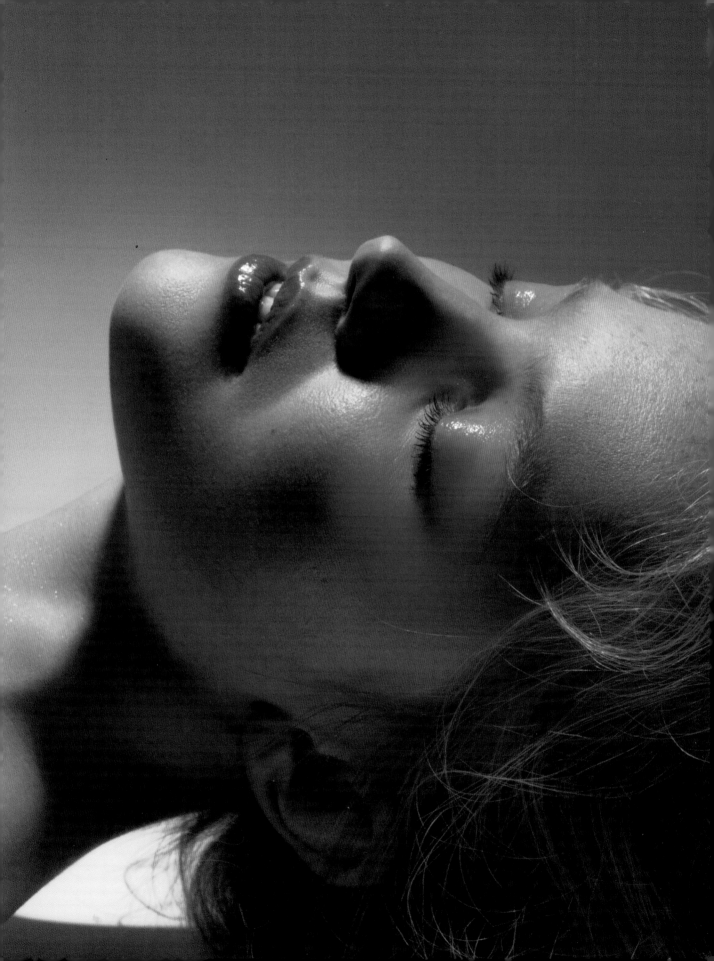

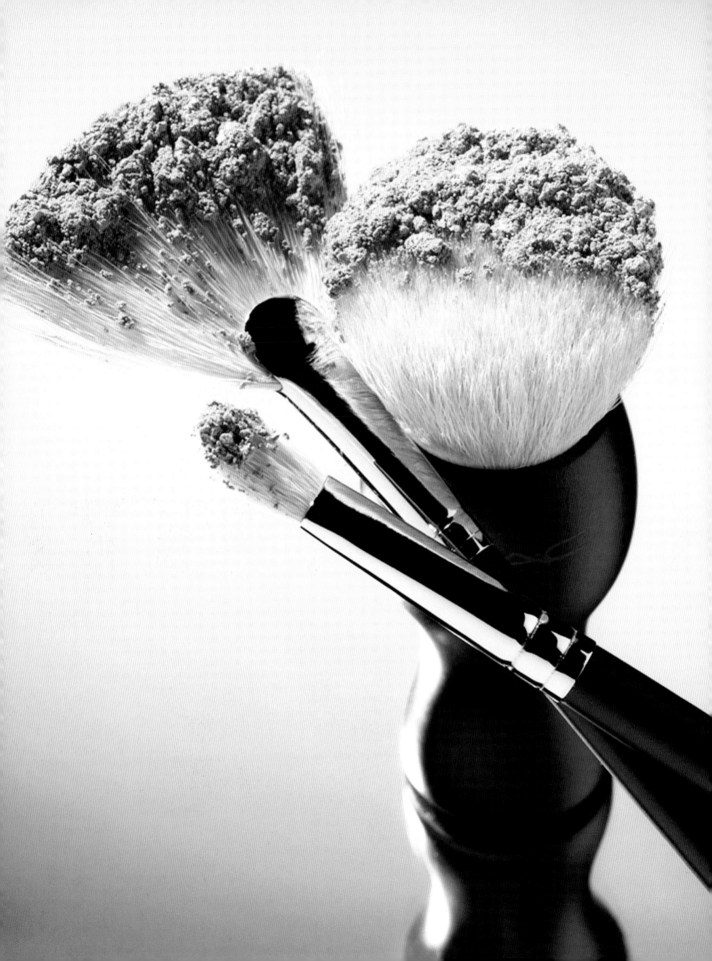

2

complexion

SAVING FACE

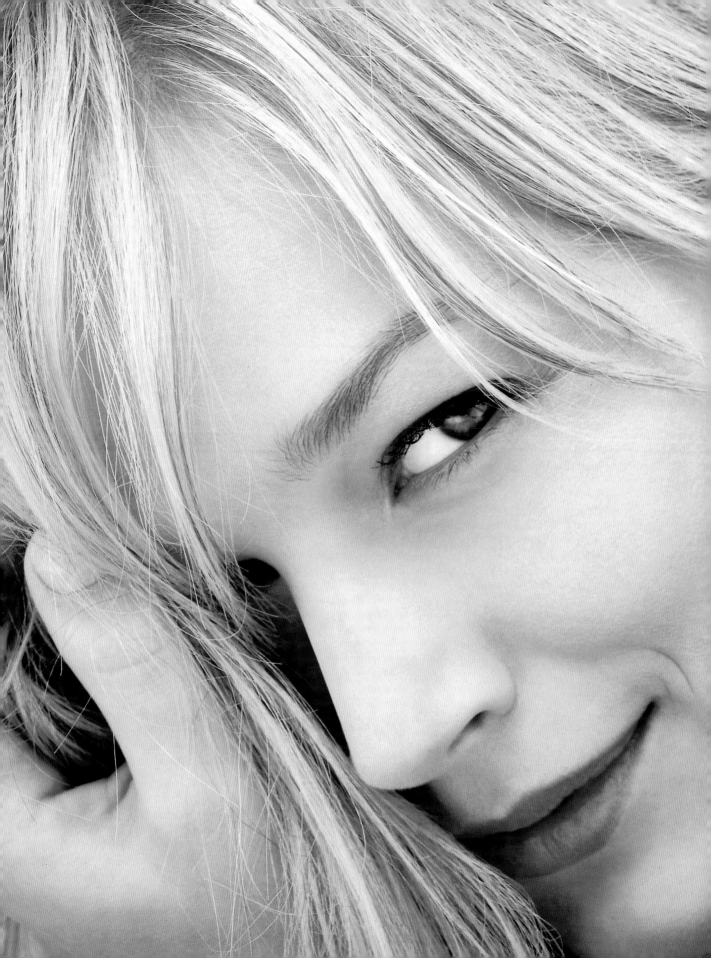

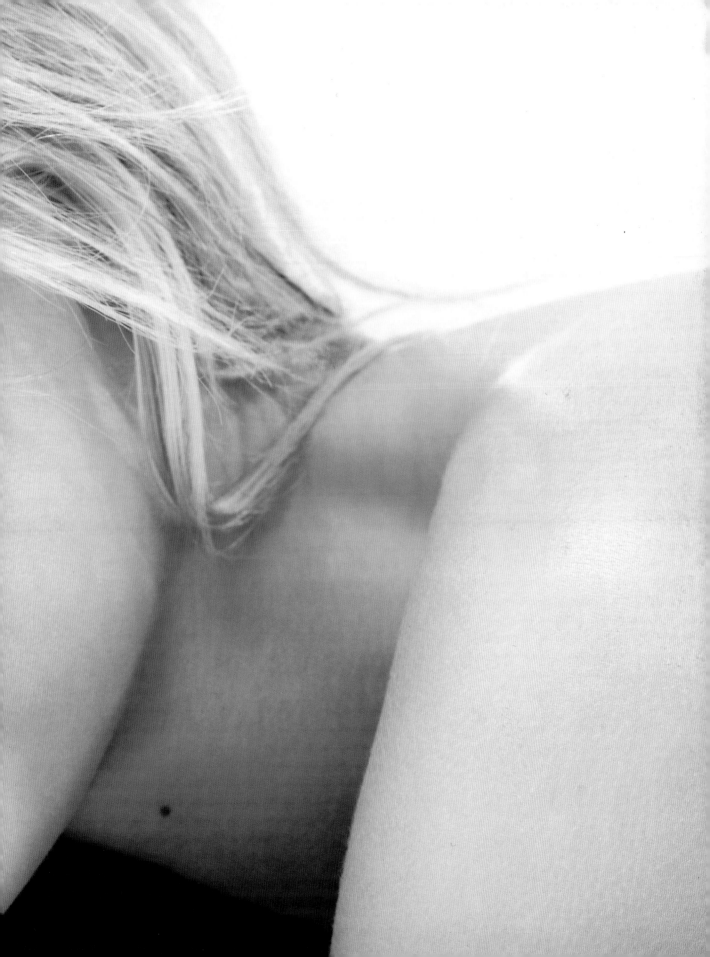

Subtle neutrals:
naturally sheer, sublimely discreet

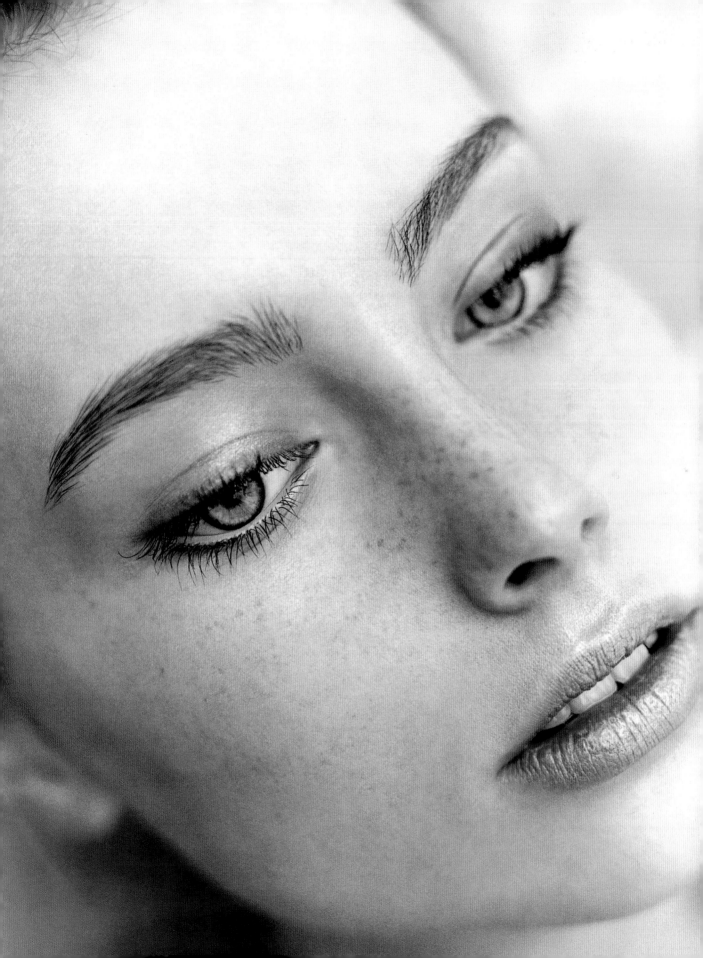

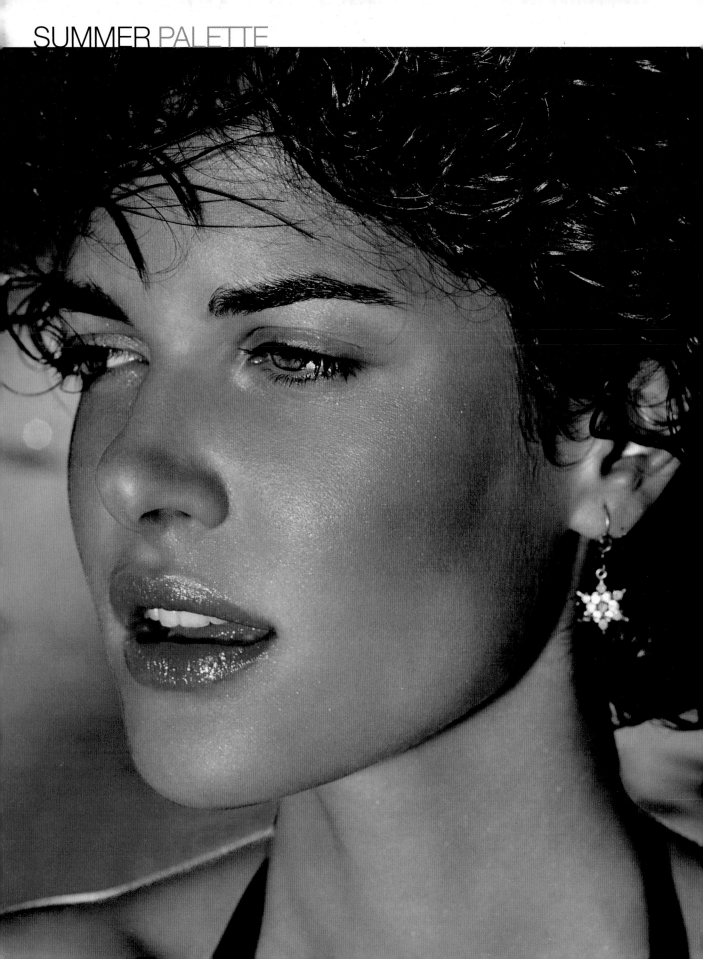

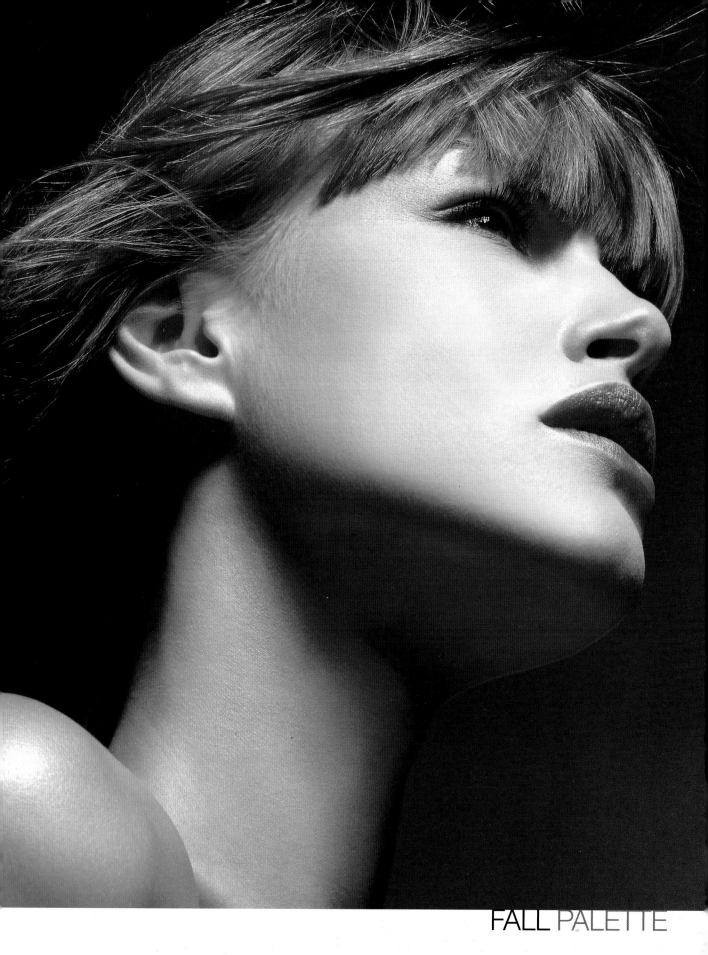

FALL PALETTE

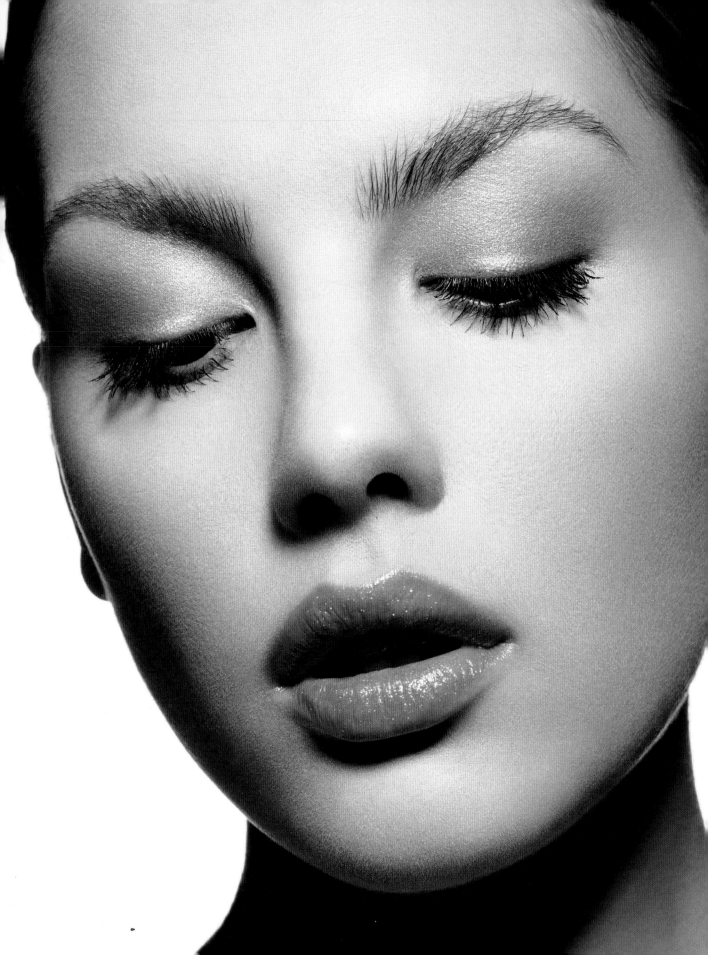

Like rose flakes and snow petals

Bare skin: The real you

Your skin dictates many of the choices you'll make surrounding makeup and other products. Knowing which of the four basic skin types is yours will help you make the right choices and keep you feeling good.

ADVICE FROM A PROFESSIONAL MAKEUP ARTIST (Stila)

Understanding your skin condition is the key. For a good self-diagnosis, closely examine your bare skin in good light. Keep one thing in mind: use your small flaws to your advantage; "blend" them in instead of trying to cover them up.

Do-at-home test

On perfectly clean skin, use a full sheet of tissue paper and apply carefully from one ear across to the other. Next, hold it up to the light and you may or may not see slightly greasy zones appear. . .

FAIR SKIN . . . normal to dry An ideally balanced pH level explains your skin's soft, supple texture. This is a precious asset that you must protect from the ravages of time and the environment. Once correctly cleansed, scrubbed, moisturized, and protected (notably from the sun's harmful rays), your face will be the perfect canvas to showcase your beauty, day in and day out.

dry to very dry Enemies of your translucent, yet ultra-sensitive and fragile, skin abound. Temperature extremes, pollution, and aging all contribute to premature wrinkles and rosacea. Your top priorities: nourish and moisturize. Eighty percent of women with this skin type don't do enough in this department. Why not try out the benefits of a humidifier?

oily This skin is generally thicker and more resistant to pollutants, damage, and even age! Your main concerns are combating shine, evening out large pores, and fighting blackheads and breakouts. Large pores can also complicate makeup application. Keep a close eye on your diet and hygiene to manage your condition.

DARK SKIN Positive factors include a high concentration of collagen and elastin (that helps curb the aging process), coupled with an acidic pH and 15 layers of sun-blocking keratin from head to toe. Makeup application and maintenance is complicated, however, by perspiration and high sebum production—the skin's natural oils.

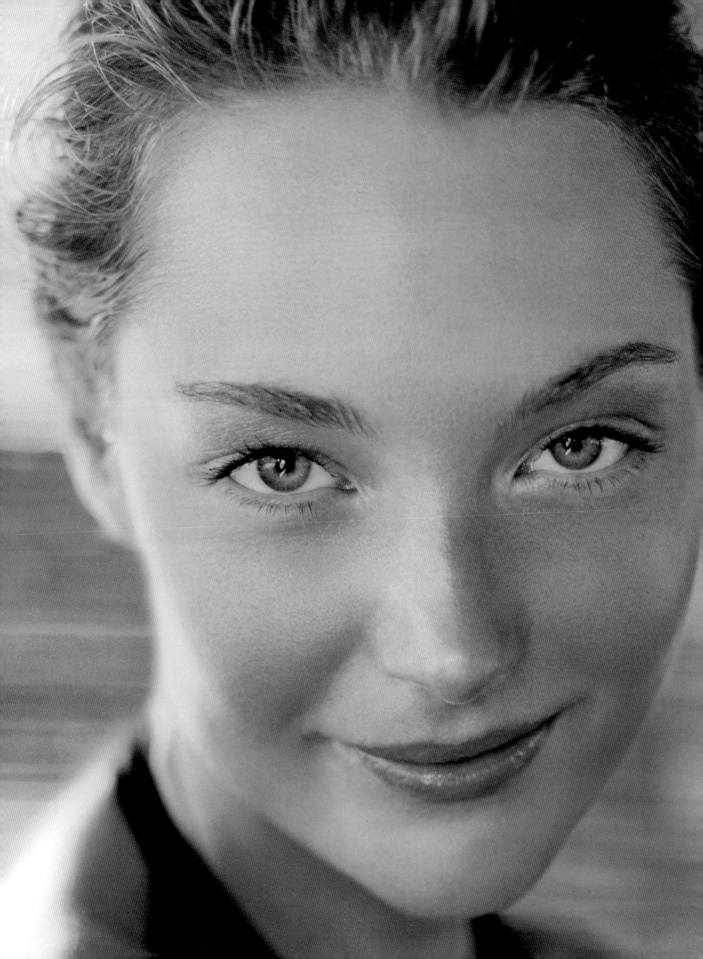

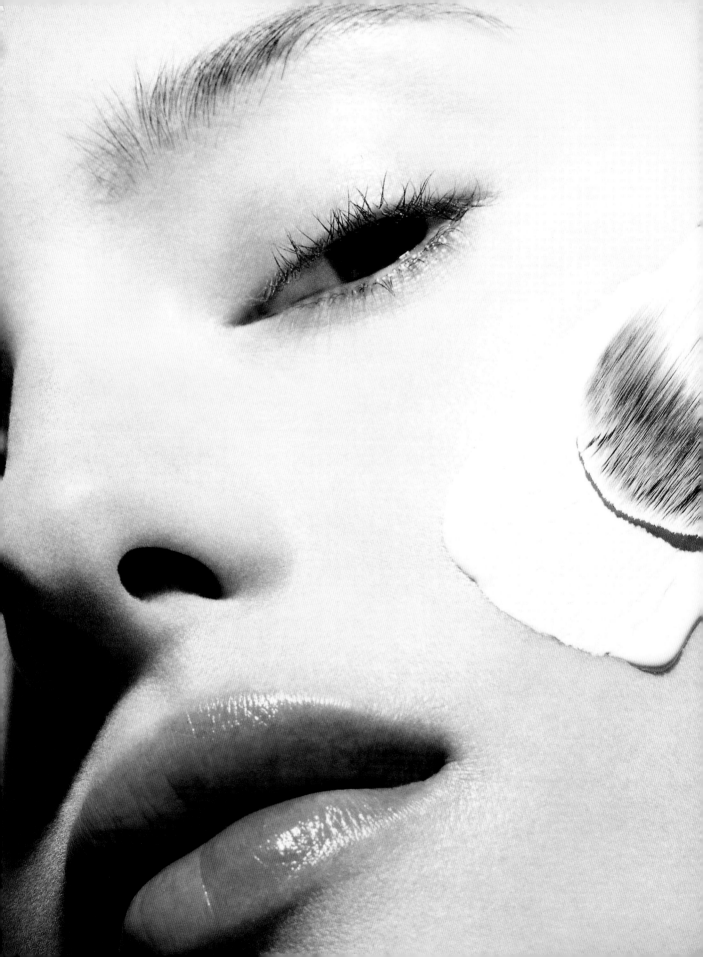

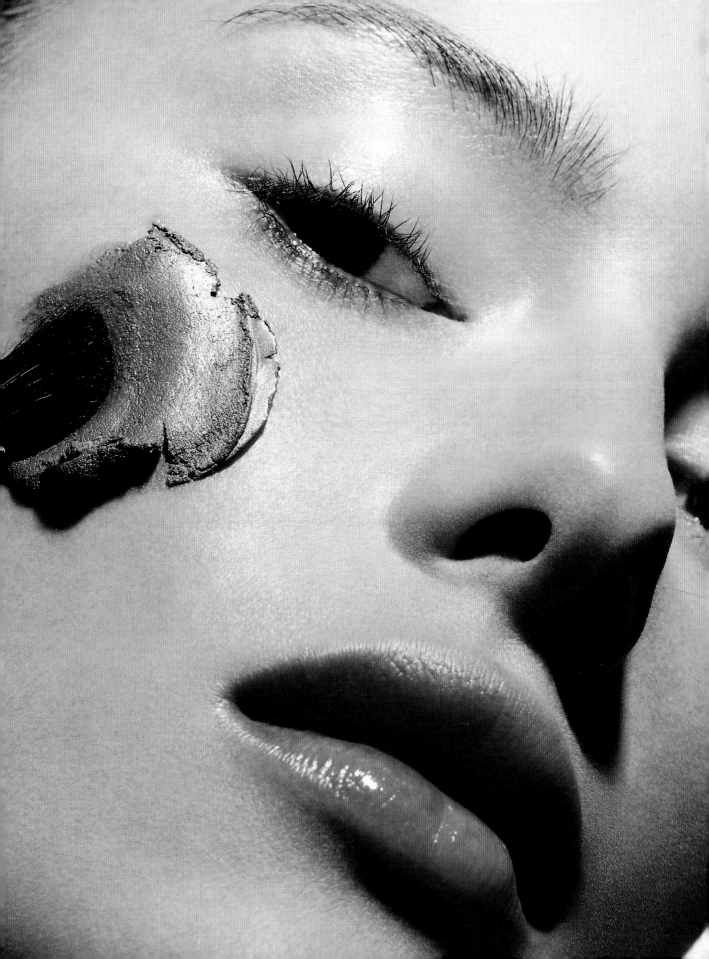

Beautiful skin
Mission: Zero flaws

You can achieve any look you want…
A canvas of impeccable skin is key.

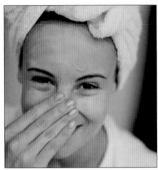

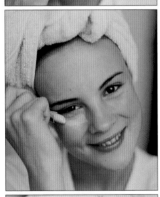

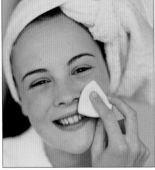

EVERY MORNING: MOISTURIZE AND PURIFY

Proper moisturizing starts with a large glass of water first thing in the morning. Even though you surely removed yesterday's makeup before going to bed, cleanse again. Use a cotton swab to clean the inner corners of your eyes and remove any traces of mascara on your lashes.

MASSAGE AND EVEN OUT

The first step to bright skin is proper preparation. Put a nickel-sized amount of lotion in the palm of your hand and perform a delicate yet vigorous massage in order to soften lines and increase the effectiveness of your moisturizer. "Warming up" your skin through circular and upward movements will help your day cream penetrate deeper and guarantee ideal moisturizing. Once microcirculation is stimulated, your skin breathes better… and it shows! Don't limit your moisturizer to your face: lavish your neck and shoulders with hydrating creams, being sure to always blend upward.

ADVICE FROM A PROFESSIONAL MAKEUP ARTIST (Stila)
Your face is a canvas that needs to be wiped clean every day. Exfoliating helps remove all the small yet toxic intruders of everyday life—climate or stress-related imperfections, dry spots, small pimples, or other blotches— and is a quick way to calm and restore your complexion.

Exfoliate once a week Using a mild exfoliant once a week is the only way to remove dead skin cells and to avoid looking ashen. Follow up with a facial.

Express Facial Envelop your face in a towel filled with ice cubes to instantly firm skin.

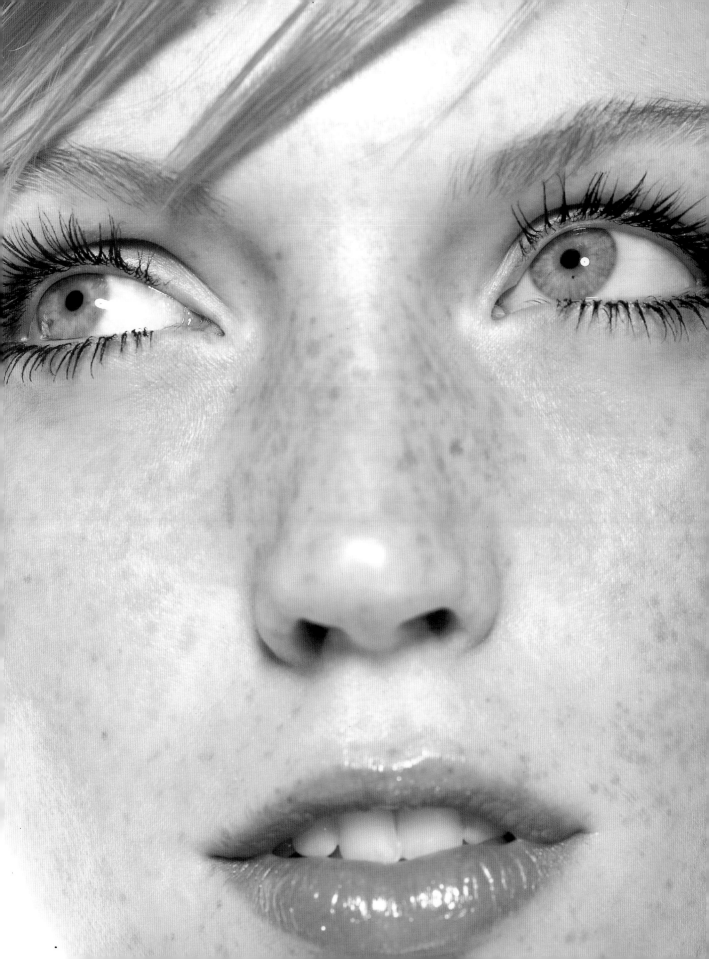

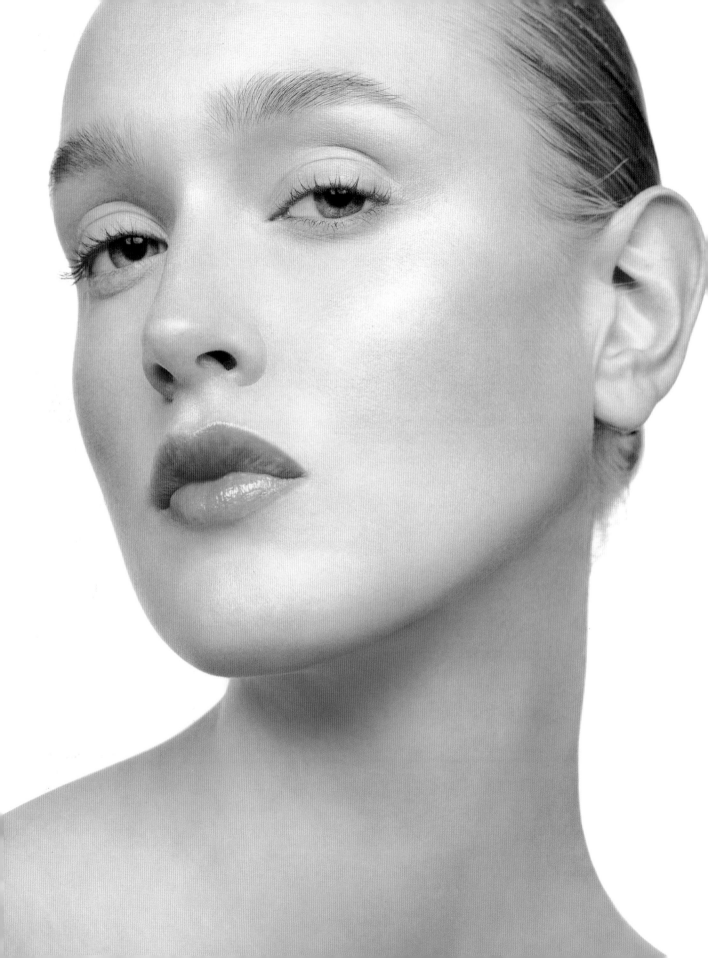

Instant glow-how

A glowing complexion has become an industry standard.

COMPLEXION ILLUMINIZERS, ENHANCERS, VEILS OF LIGHT... These are to skin what gloss is to lips, a new generation of products that brilliantly keep their promise: they contain pearly pigments that reflect and diffuse light to give your skin a radiant glow and make it anything but lackluster.

USE alone, or for more spectacular effects, couple it with a classic foundation—the two can be easily blended if their respective consistency allows. The result is a perfectly luminous base.

CHOOSE beige tones for pale complexions or muted apricot tones for more golden skin. Place a dot on the back of your hand and pass the brush through it before applying a very small amount to the middle of your eyelid, the bridge of your nose, and the top of your cheekbones. It will capture the light, and your skin will be radiant as a result.

FOR MAXIMUM LUSTER you can also use it after foundation, for a final touch, on your cheekbones, nose, chin, brow bone, and your hairline.

To plump your lips and hold lipstick in place: blend up to the lip line before applying lip color.

What you'll need
- a full brush
- nimble fingers!

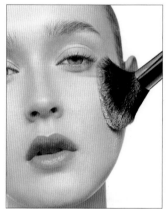

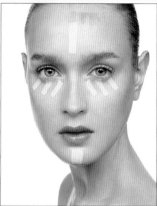

The magic line: center of the forehead, bridge of the nose, tip of the chin, and top of the cheekbones

A no-stress guide to concealer

A know-it-all product that does it all: hides, disguises, and corrects. It's impossible to live without, but how do you find the one that's right for you?

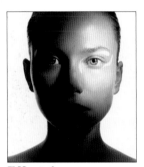

Effect 1
Light up your face.

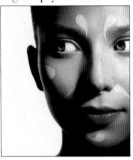

Effect 2
Highlight your features.

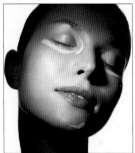

Effect 3
Hide imperfections.

THE RIGHT COLOR Concealer must be perfectly identical to your skin tone. The name of the game is absolute uniformity—flawless blending with your natural skin color.

IN THE BAG...OR NOT Whether or not you have dark circles under your eyes, concealer smoothes the skin, diminishes wrinkles, erases blood vessels along your nose, and brightens your eyes at their inner corners or on the tops of your eyelids.

Concealer also covers pimples and softens the lines between your eyebrows. It adds radiance to your smile at the corners of your mouth and reduces shine on the tip of your nose.

APPLY with vertical sweeps aided by small patting motions, using a small brush—an easily procurable tool of the pros—for blending.

How to cover a pimple Use concealer a half shade lighter than your skin. Apply directly on the pimple, and don't forget to use powder to keep the product in place.

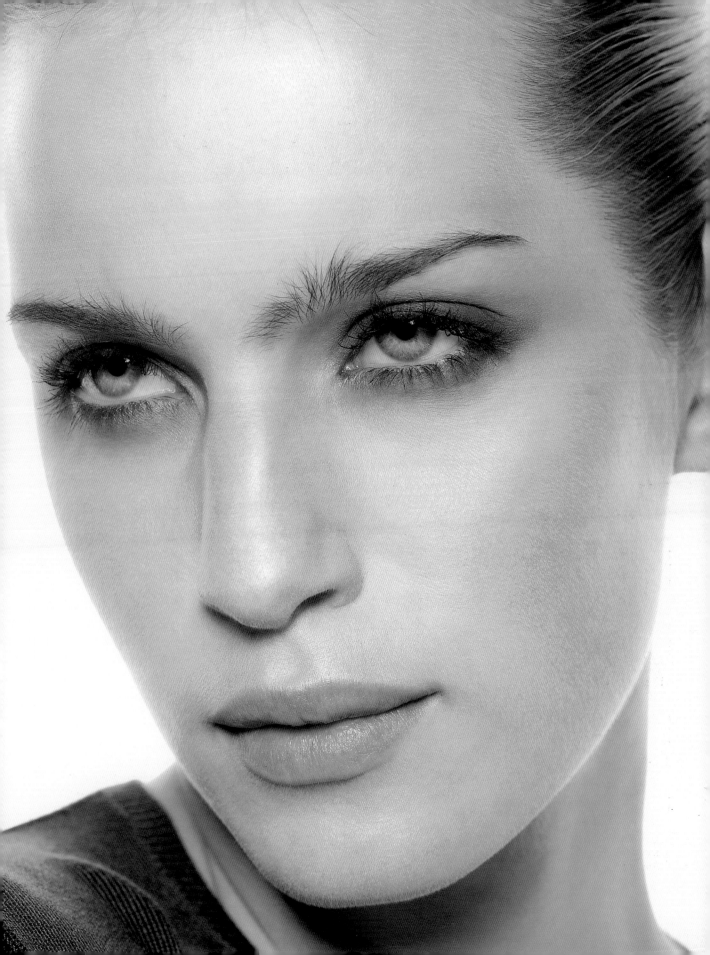

Ace your base

*Mastering the art of blending formulas and textures
to silky smoothness for just the right subtle shade.
Foundation is not what it used to be!*

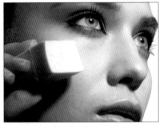

Freshness tip: Use a damp
latex makeup sponge to blend
your foundation.

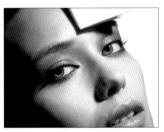

Beware of the T-Zone!
To avoid shine, gently pat
your forehead, the bridge of
your nose, and your chin
with a tissue.

For dry skin, you need a rich and satiny foundation. If your skin is oily, you'll need something lighter and smoother with a matte finish. Today's foundations moisturize and protect while still letting skin breathe, and some even have anti-aging properties.

Test **SHADES** along your jawline and opt for one tone lighter than your skin. Aim for unifying your complexion, not changing it. You don't want to run the risk of unsightly streaks.

If you use your **FINGERTIPS** to apply foundation, use a massaging motion to tone, perfect, and smoothly blend into your skin.

When using a dry **FLAT BRUSH** (the fuller the brush, the easier the application) or a slightly damp **MAKEUP SPONGE,** it's important to lightly pat the foundation on. Pay close attention to the contours of your eyes where buildup can lead to one bad effect of poor application: accentuated wrinkles. Apply, starting in the center of your face, and blend outward for the best effect.

**ADVICE FROM A
PROFESSIONAL
MAKEUP ARTIST
(Stila)**
Choose your makeup according to the texture of your skin—we like certain formulas just as we like certain drinks; we know what feels good. To get a "feeling" for a particular product, place a small amount on the back of your hand and warm it up with your fingertips before applying it to your face.

Tip for longer hold
Spraying water through
a tissue will fix your
foundation.

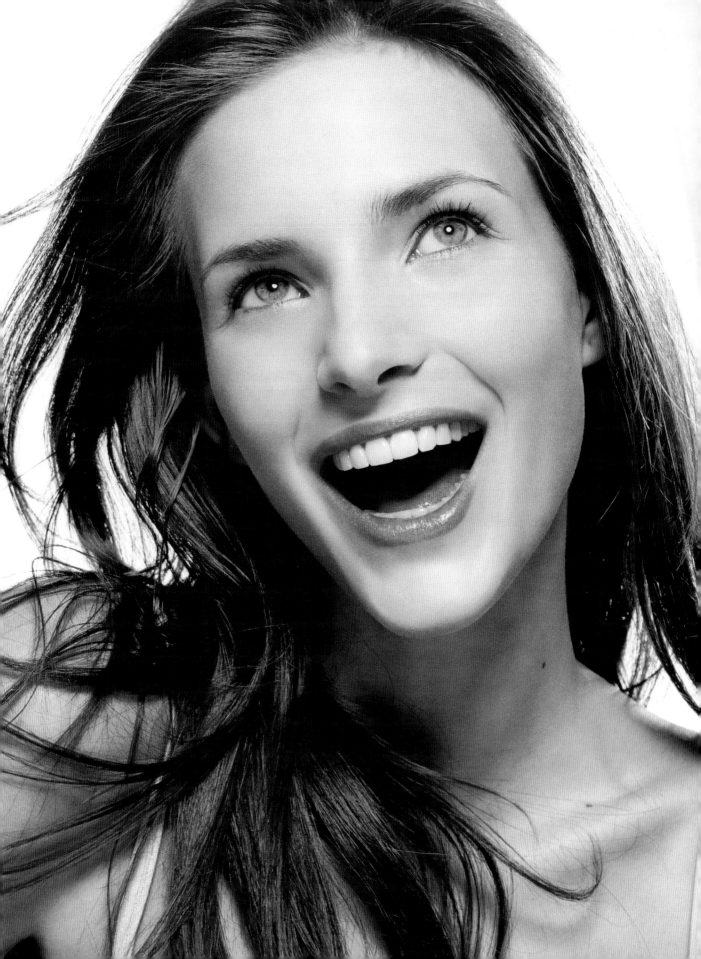

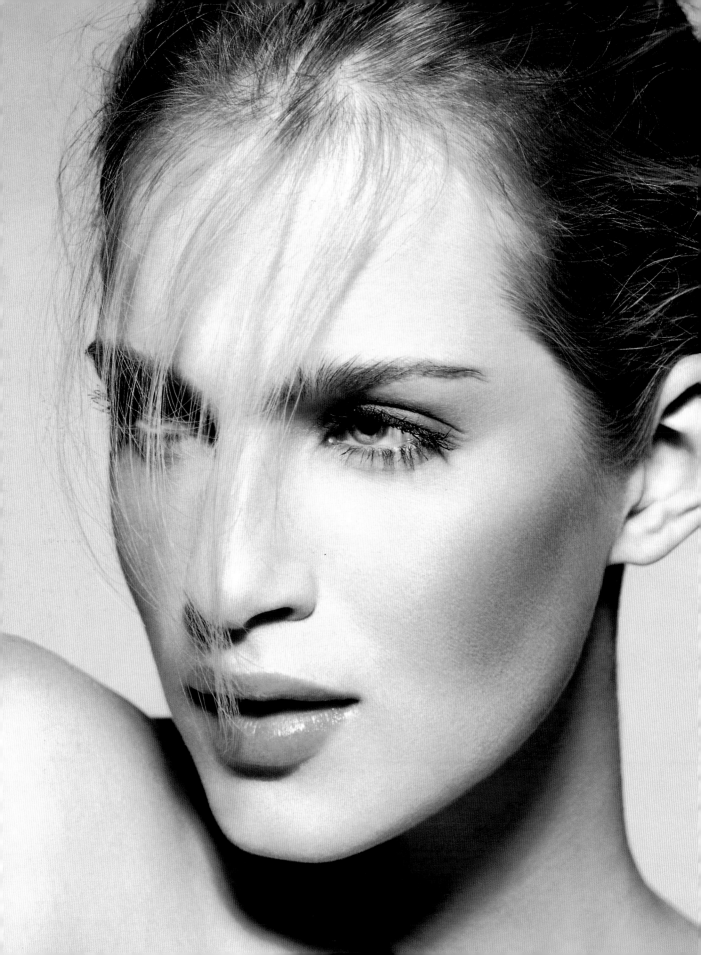

Bluff with blush

Blush is the final touch for getting your face in place.

LOCATION IS EVERYTHING and the shape of your face is your guide. You can sculpt round cheeks (start at the top of your ear, and work your way down in a crescent motion until below your cheekbones), soften a square-like appearance (apply close to the ear and blend toward the cheekbones), or counter a rectangular facial structure (apply horizontally on cheekbones).

COLOR CODES Fair-skinned women should use lively pinks and reds. Darker-skinned women should opt for browns and corals. Tender roses, on the other hand, suit everyone!

To ensure effective blending, your **BRUSH** should not be too full.

Your **FINGERTIPS** can be used with mousse or cream formulas that become powdery after application. Dab the product on with your index finger for the right amount, and blend from your jaw to your cheekbone.

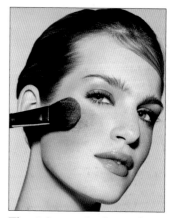

The right powder brings light to your eyelids and adds radiance to your face.

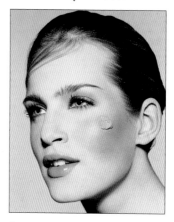

Cream-to-powder blush lets you sculpt your cheekbones with your fingertips.

What you'll need:
- blush brush
- cream blush
- powder blush

Bottled bronzing

Self-tanners are both the most flattering and the most dangerous of inventions. Using them requires a bit of skill!

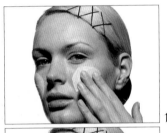

1

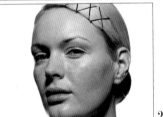

2

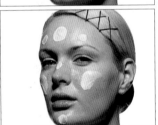

3

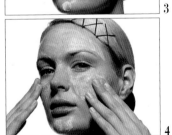

4

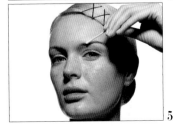

5

1 FOR A PERFECTLY UNIFORM TAN, always start fresh: make sure you've used a gentle exfoliant (chemical or mechanical) to remove all dead skin cells.

2 WELL-MOISTURIZED SKIN is even more important when self-tanning since DHA (the principal component of self-tanners) has a tendency to dry skin out by draining water from skin cells.

3 APPLY SMALL AMOUNTS to your forehead, cheeks, and chin—all the places the sun would hit first—without forgetting your ears and neck, blending toward your shoulders.

4 SPREAD self-tanners uniformly but quickly across your face by massaging with the flats of your fingers. Immediately wash your hands (and nails) vigorously with soap and water.

5 TO AVOID AN ORANGY LOOK immediately after application wipe a cotton swab or a damp paper towel across your eyebrows and along your hairline.

ADVICE FROM ALINE SCHMITT (studio makeup artist)
Wait 15 minutes before applying makeup after using a self-tanner. Your foundation will tone down while your self-tanner kicks in!

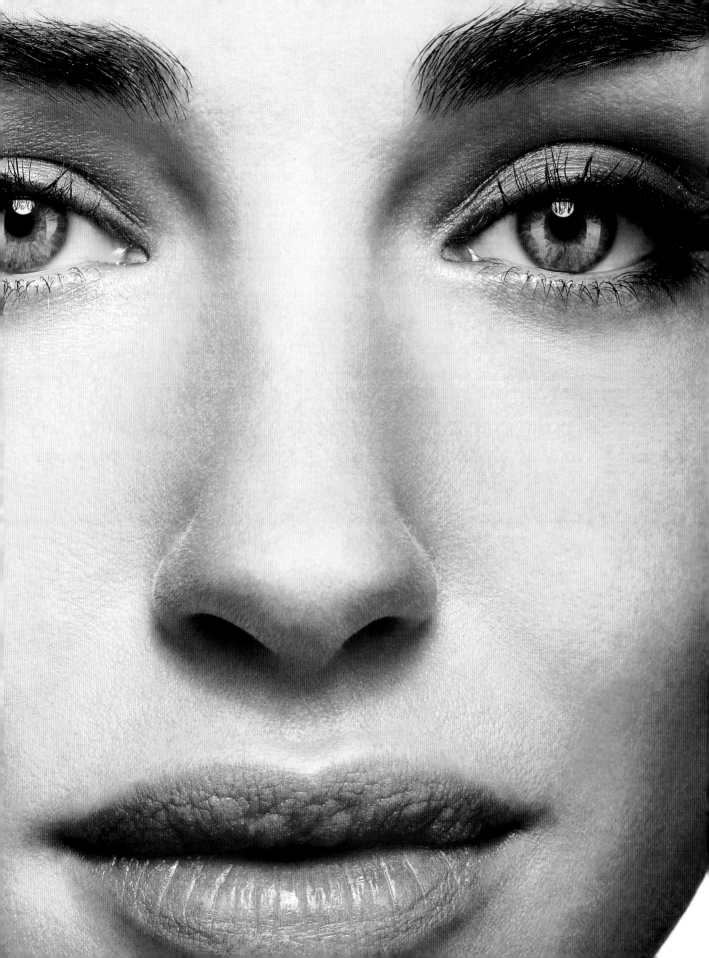

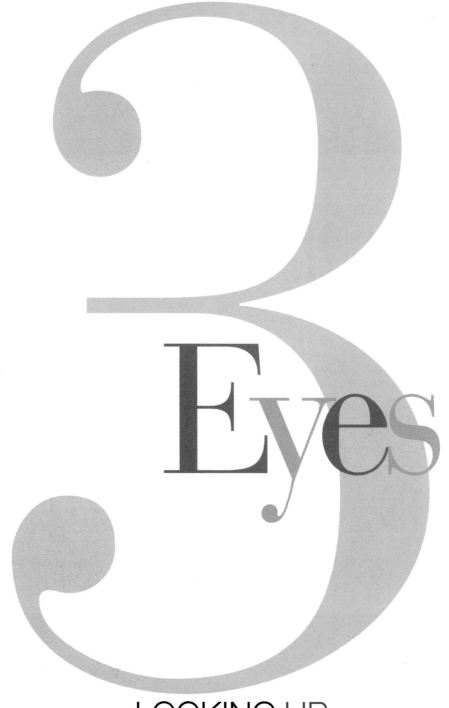

3 Eyes

LOOKING UP

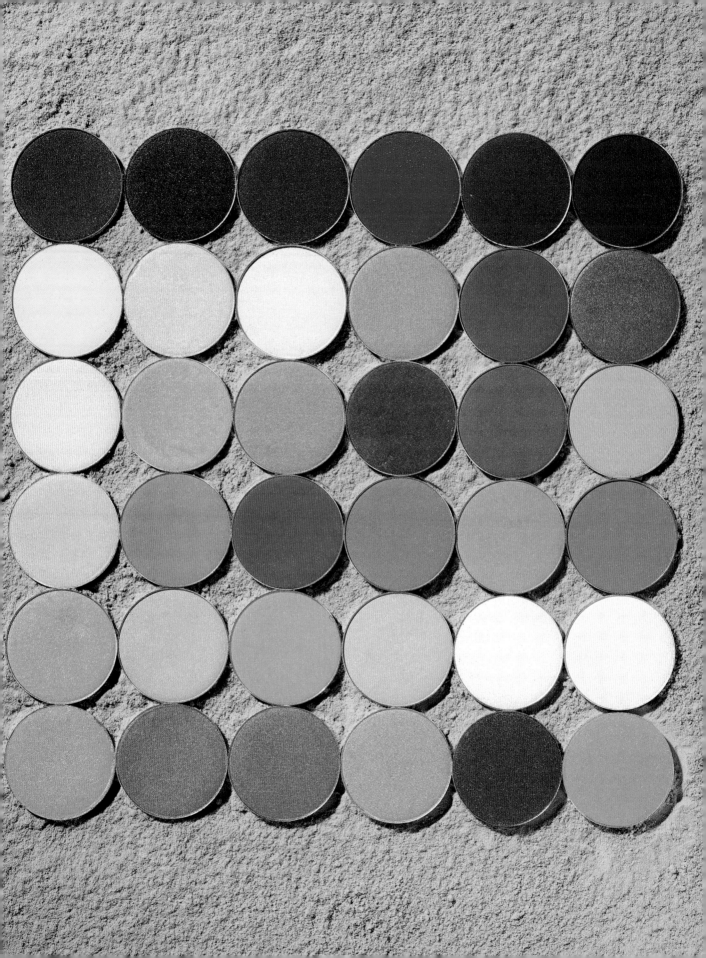

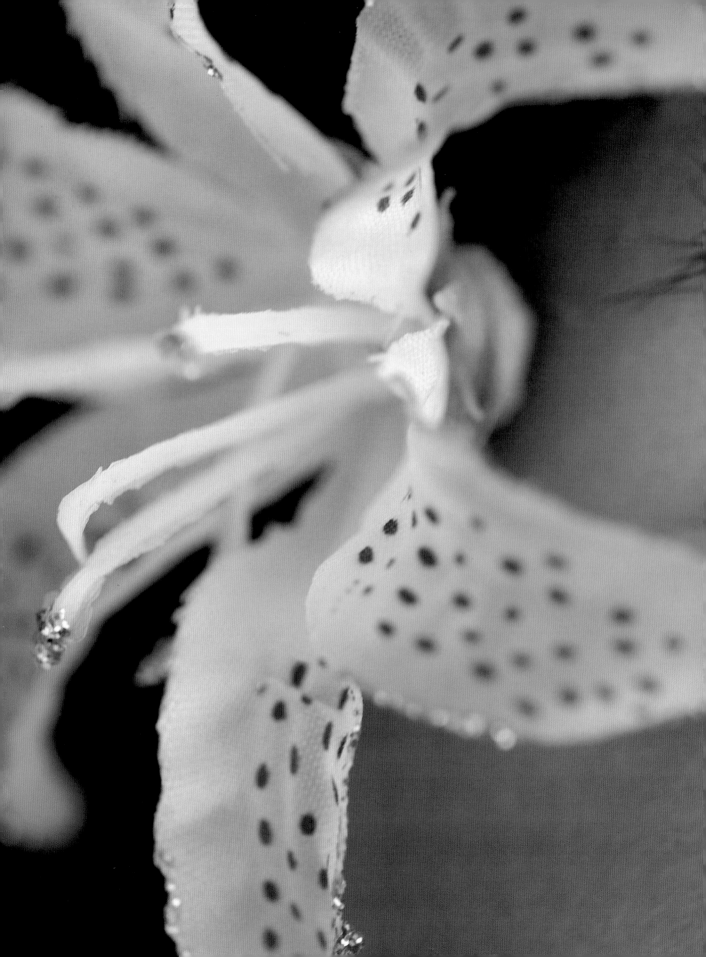

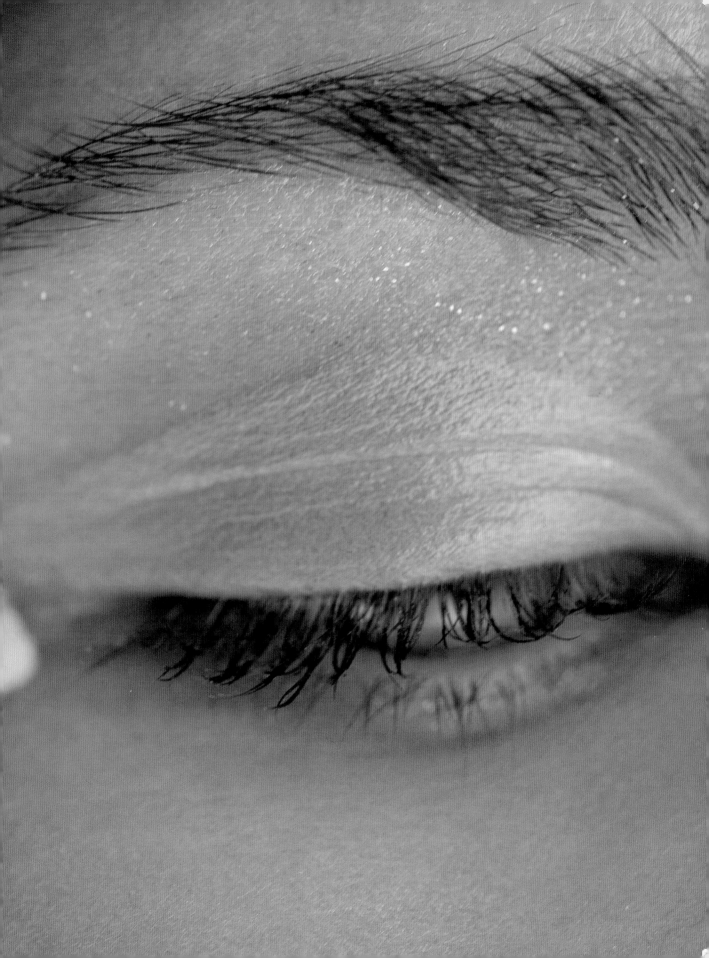

Audacious as hope mysterious as emeralds A shimmering Green sheen

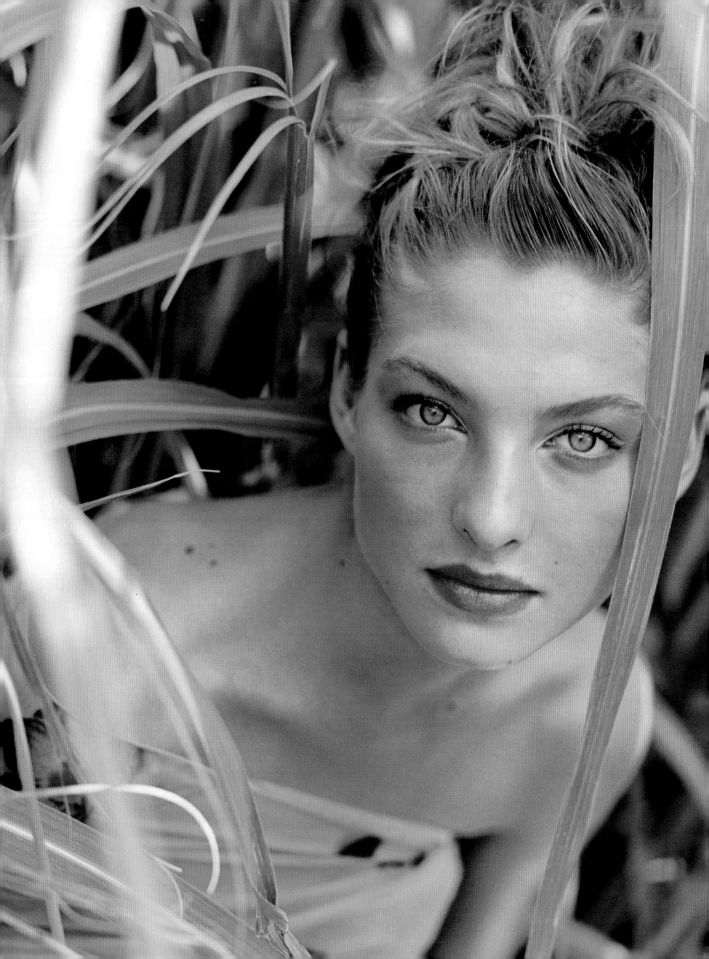

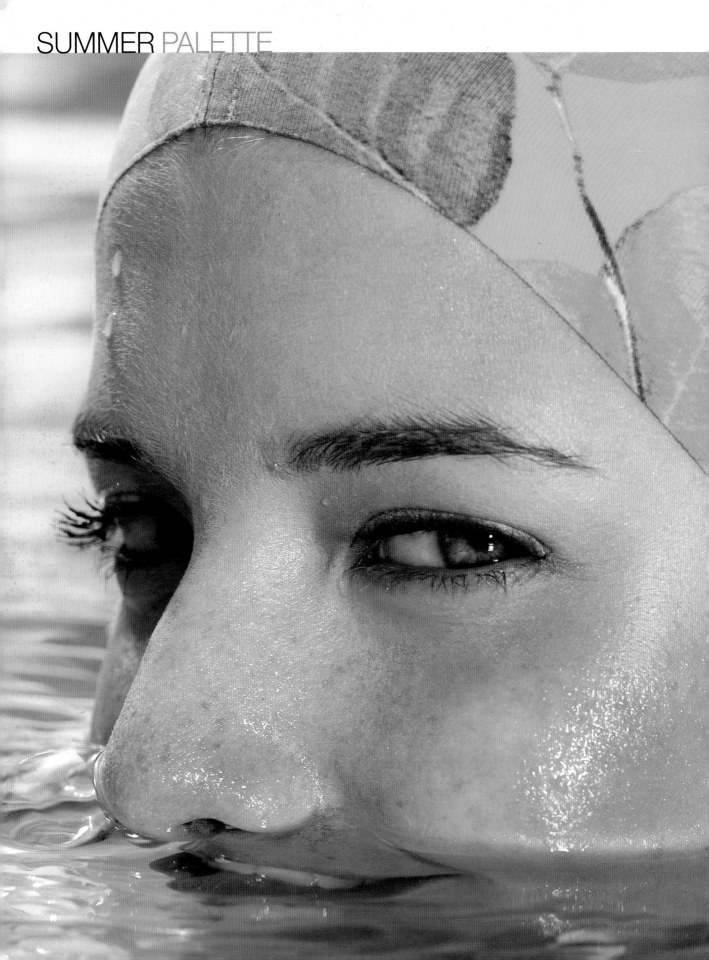

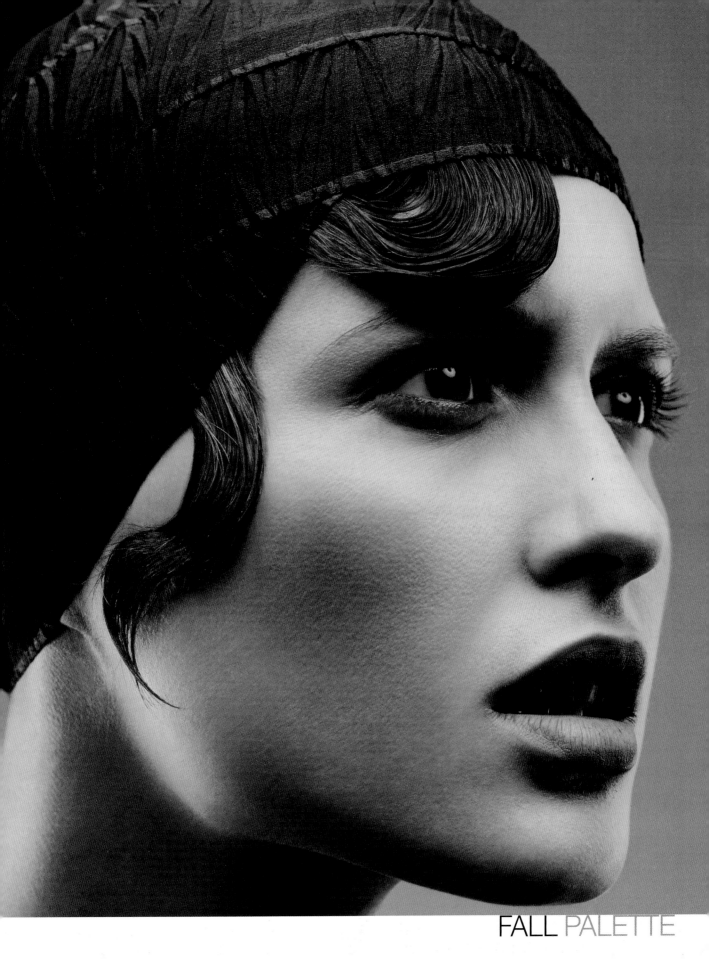

FALL PALETTE

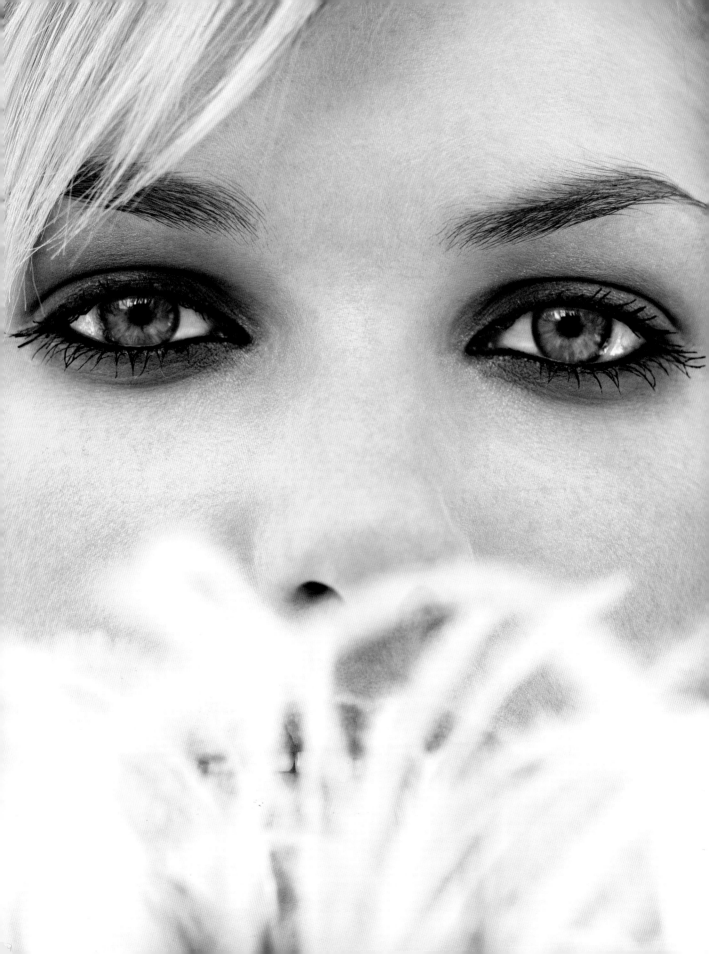

Intense gaze and pale frost, there's fire under the ice.

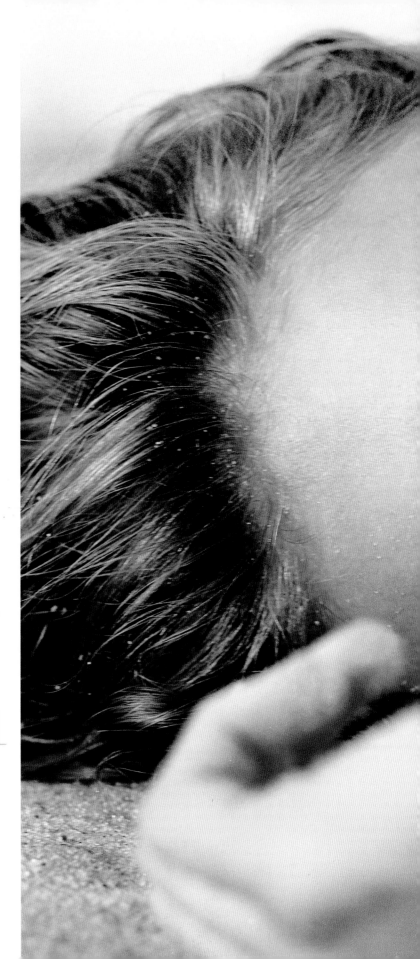

A cocktail
of ocean
blue and
marine
green
for a
Technicolor
siren

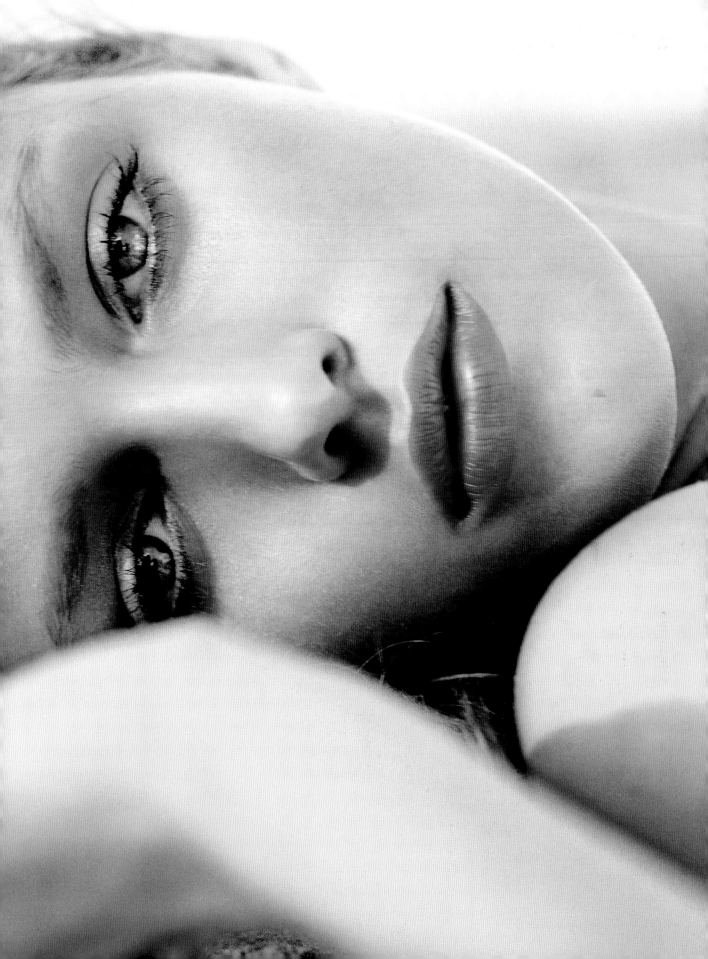

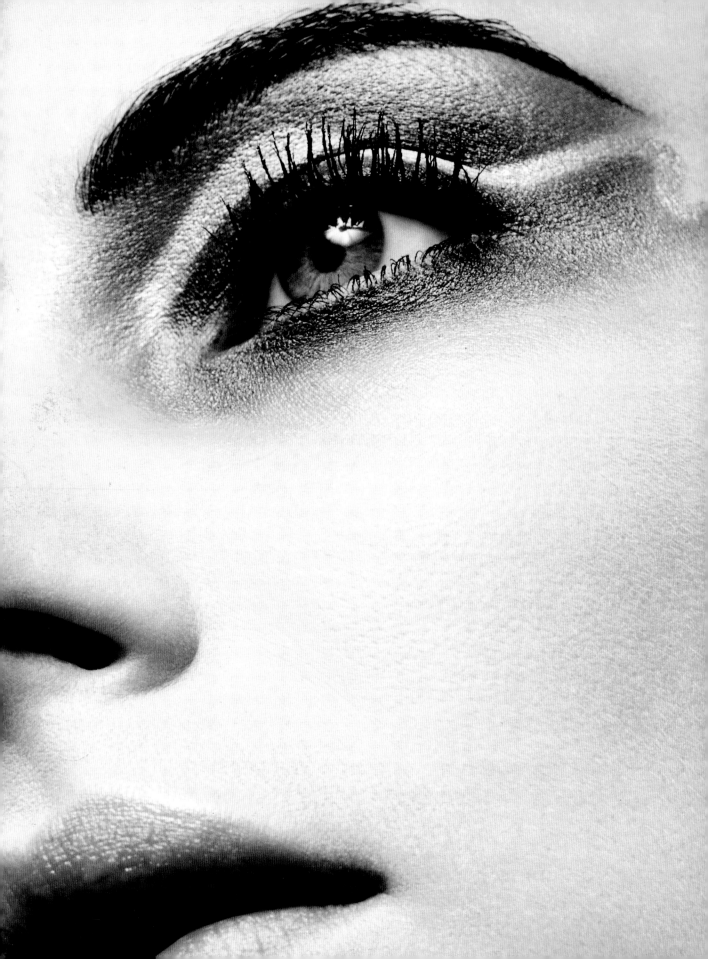

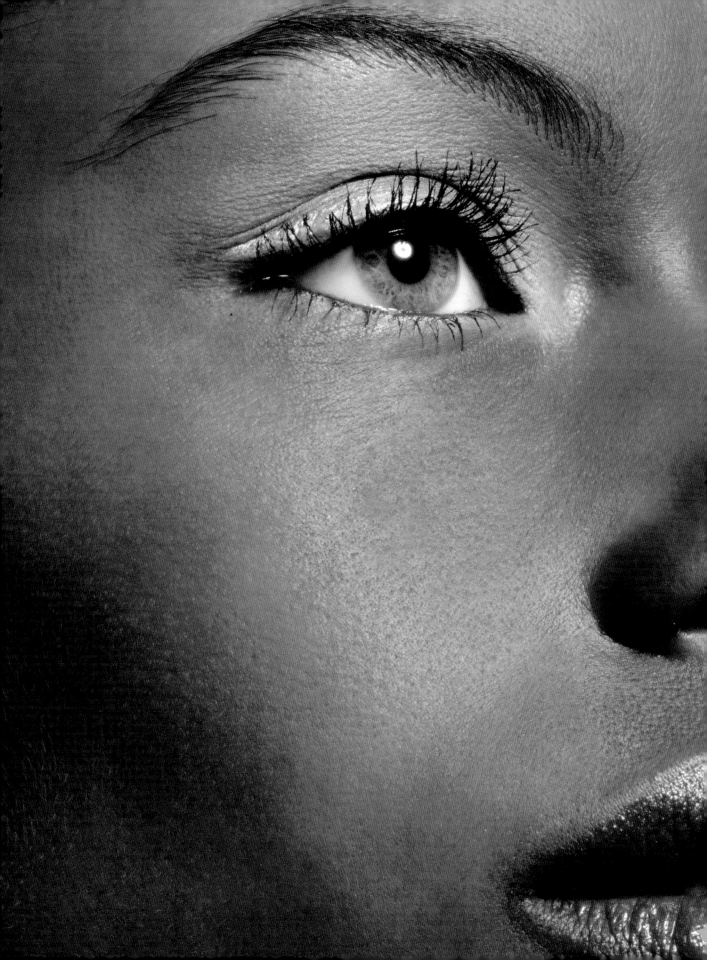

Drawing the line

There's nothing easier than a swipe of eyeliner to bring out your personality. Here are some simple tips to help you keep your eye on the ball.

CHOOSE YOUR WEAPON To find the right pencil for you, test some on the back of your hand. If a pencil is too dry, it won't leave as much color as you'd like, and you may have to press down too much to apply it. On the other hand, if it's too soft, the color will undoubtedly smudge. For maximum precision, look for a soft yet firm tip that you can smudge if desired.

COLOR CONSCIOUS The possibilities are limitless, with tints for every occasion: from matte to shimmery and from muted to pearly, eyeliner can add unbelievable depth to your eyes. Sober dark tones will add fire to blue and green irises but will bring out the gold in hazels and dark browns.

A TIP FROM TERRY (BY TERRY)
To ensure maximum hold, gently stretch and hold your eyelid closed with a finger while applying pencil across the whole lid.

A thin line drawn on the bottom lid—just above the lashes of your lower inner eyelid—will really make your eyes look bigger and doe-shaped.

What you'll need
Be sure to buy a special sharpener intended only for your eye pencils. A regular pencil sharpener is poorly suited for the task and is not very hygienic.

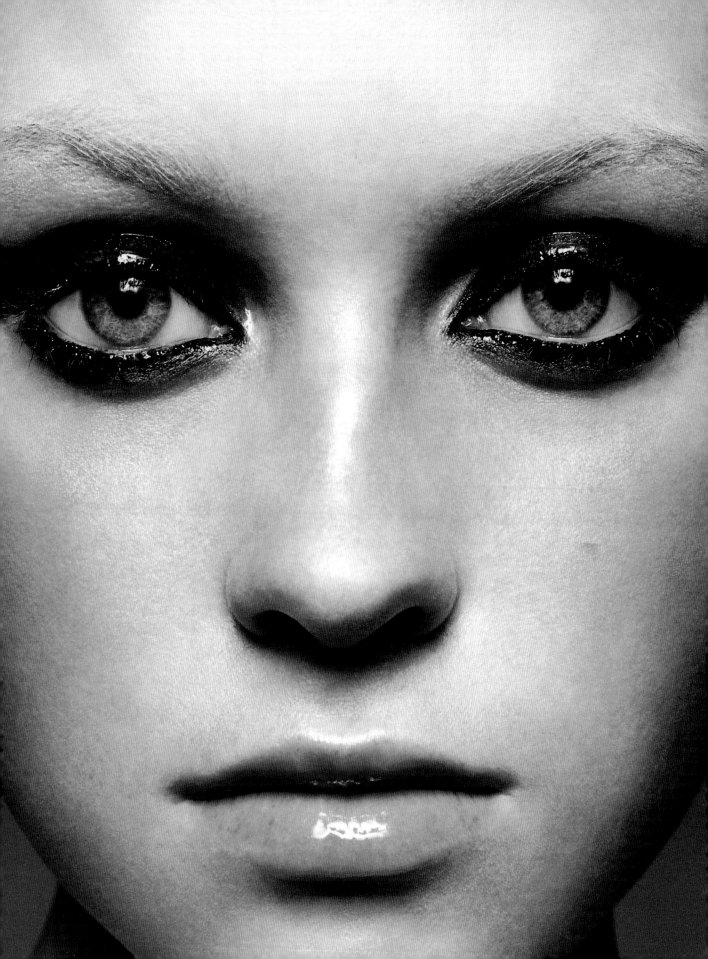

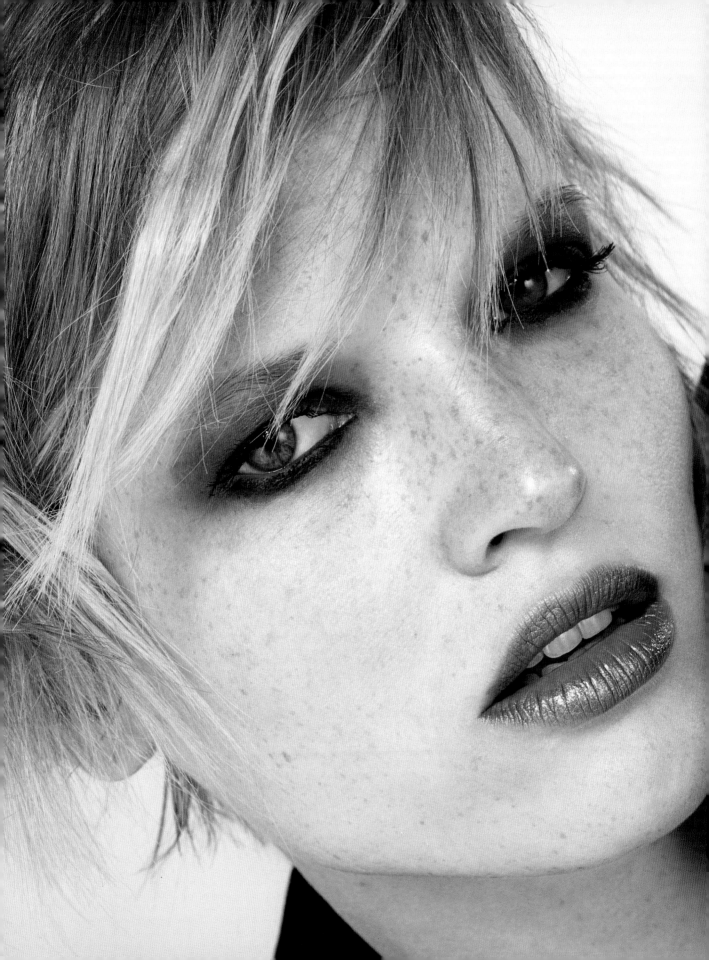

Pencil me in

The art of eye definition.

KOHL PENCILS should be warmed up first with your hand (or a light bulb): the color effect on your lids will be even more dramatic. Apply between your lashes for greater depth. Lightly pulling on the tip of your eyelid will help draw color underneath. Smudge with a brush, but beware of closing off the outer corner: this can result in a too-heavy look.

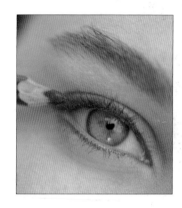

KEEPING A LID ON SHADOWS Starting from the bottom of your lashes, use a zigzag movement for blending. To achieve an understated look, smudge a bit with your fingertip (you can use a dot of your eye concealer) or a pencil. Hold your eyelid while applying for maximum definition, and don't be afraid to run over a bit at the top which can give your eyes a younger look.

TIPS & TRICKS: FIX YOUR FLAWS

Separate close-set eyes Use a lighter pencil from the inner corner to the middle of your eye, then finish off with a darker tone at the outer edges.

Perk up droopy eyes Start with a darker color at the inner eye, then finish off with something lighter.

ADVICE FROM TERRY (by Terry)
A bright spot of light and cool mauve shadow around your eye will brighten things up and make your eyes look more rested.

In the line of sight: Just one aim. . . looking gorgeous

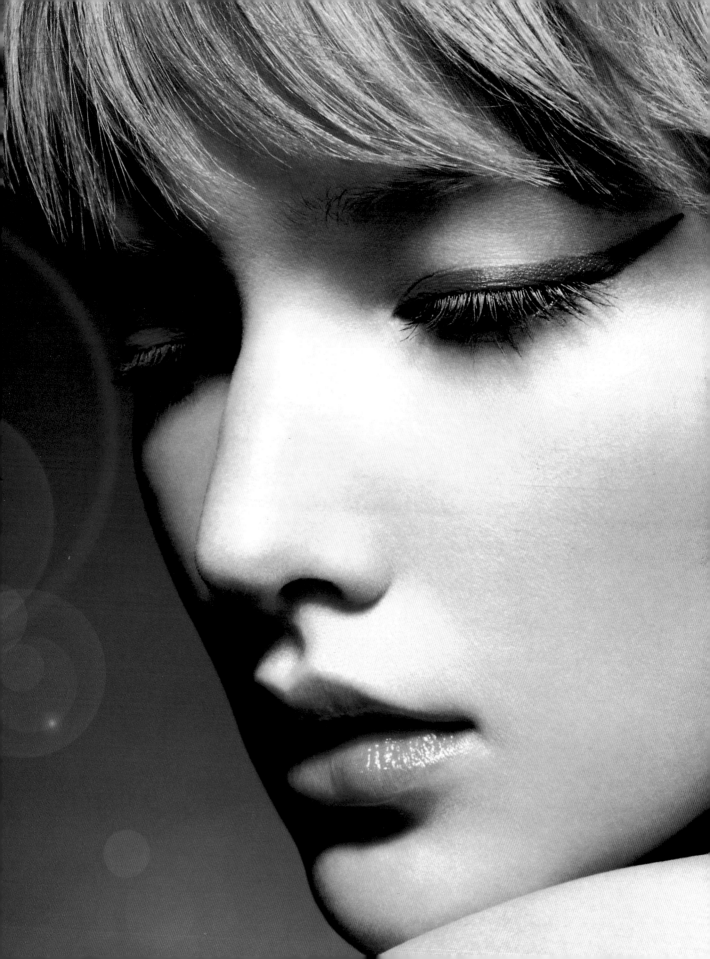

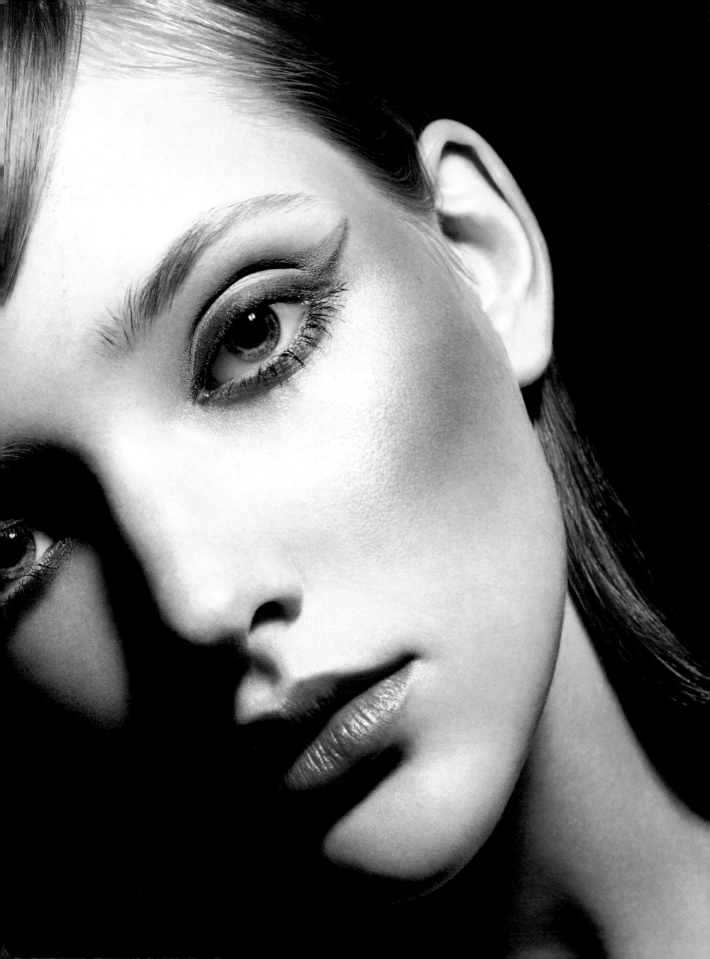

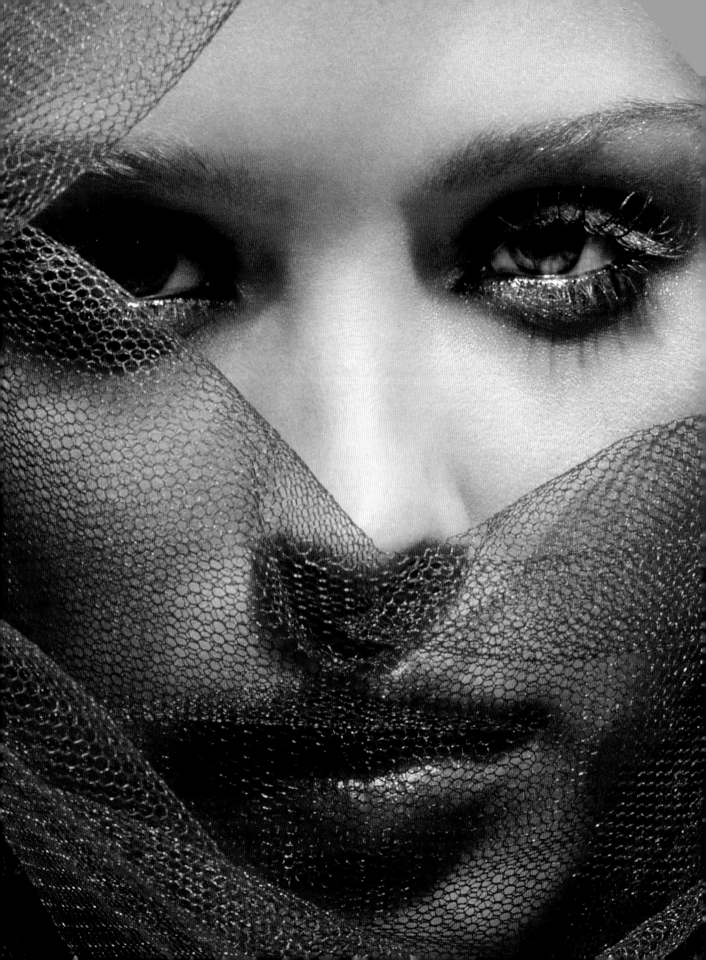

Give 'em an eyeful

It's a comeback for the makeup star of the seventies: new liquid and gel eyeliners.

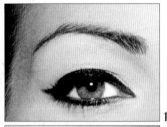

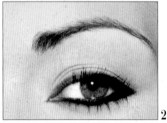

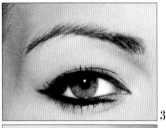

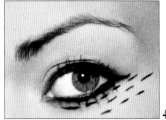

1 **DOE, A DEER** **Upper lid** To prevent uncontrolled excess, firmly hold your lid with one finger while applying eyeliner from the inner corner. Work gradually toward the middle, thickening as desired, and then tapering toward the outer corner. Be sure that both lines are equal. **Lower lid** Same principle—start with a thin line that thickens toward the outer corner.

2 **MATCHING TONES** **Upper lid** For guaranteed elegance, overlap shades of subtly smudged eyeshadows with the lightest tones on top, and complete the look with thin eyeliner matching your iris. **Lower lid** A broad stroke that softly runs over into the inner eyelid will give your gaze immediate intensity.

3 **OPTICAL ILLUSIONS** Enlarge your eyes by accentuating your upper eyelid: start from the inner corner and aim for your ear. **To correct a "droopy" look,** highlight your lower lid by working away from the eyelash line as you get closer to your nose.

4 **HAUTE COUTURE** A bold choice that will also bring out your personality and your creativity!

ADVICE FROM PATRICK LORENTZ (Estée Lauder) Always pick a thin and supple eyeliner brush, and don't put too much liner on it: this is the best way to prevent smearing and runs.

Top stitch = Top glamour? The look on the opposite page is achieved with the flat end of the brush. Keep your skin taut while applying by placing your finger just above your cheekbones and lightly pulling downwards.

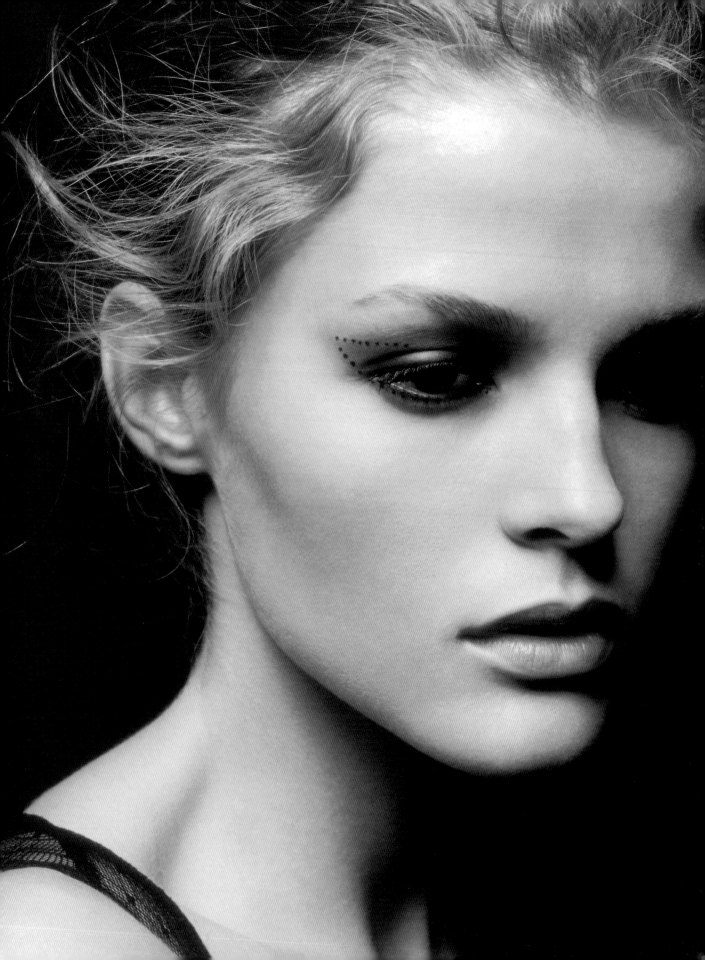

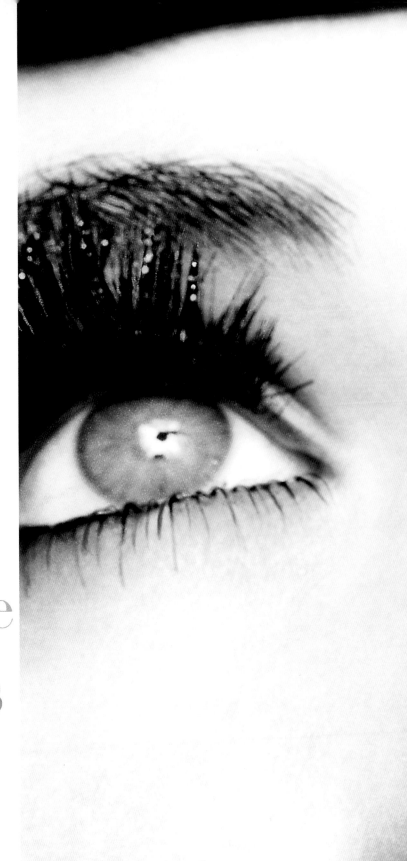

Eyelashes—
a sublime
gateway
to dreams
and
emotions

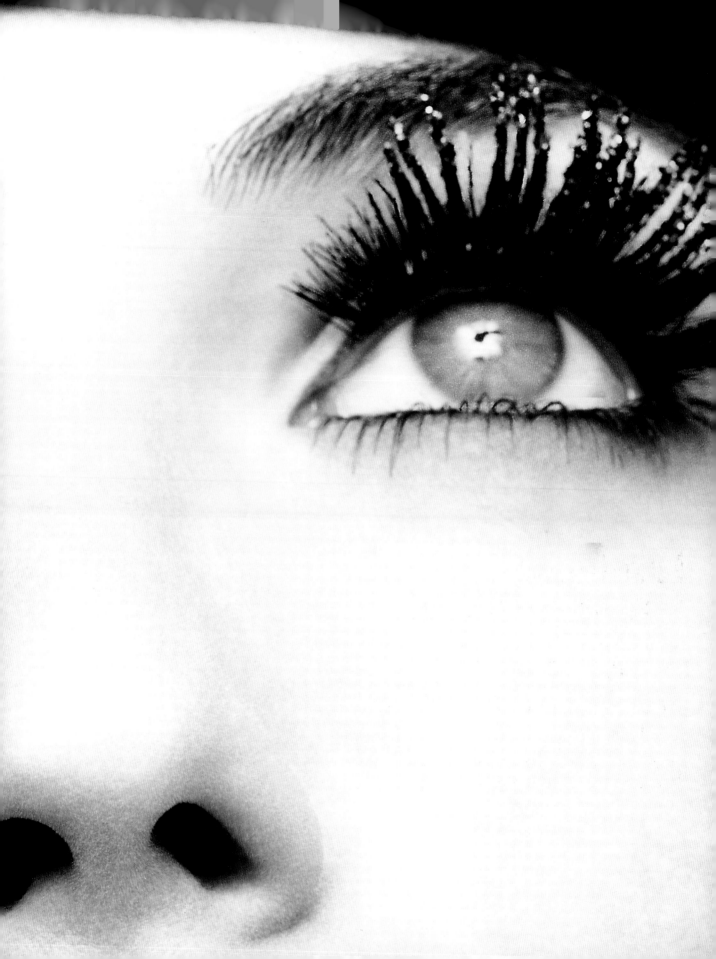

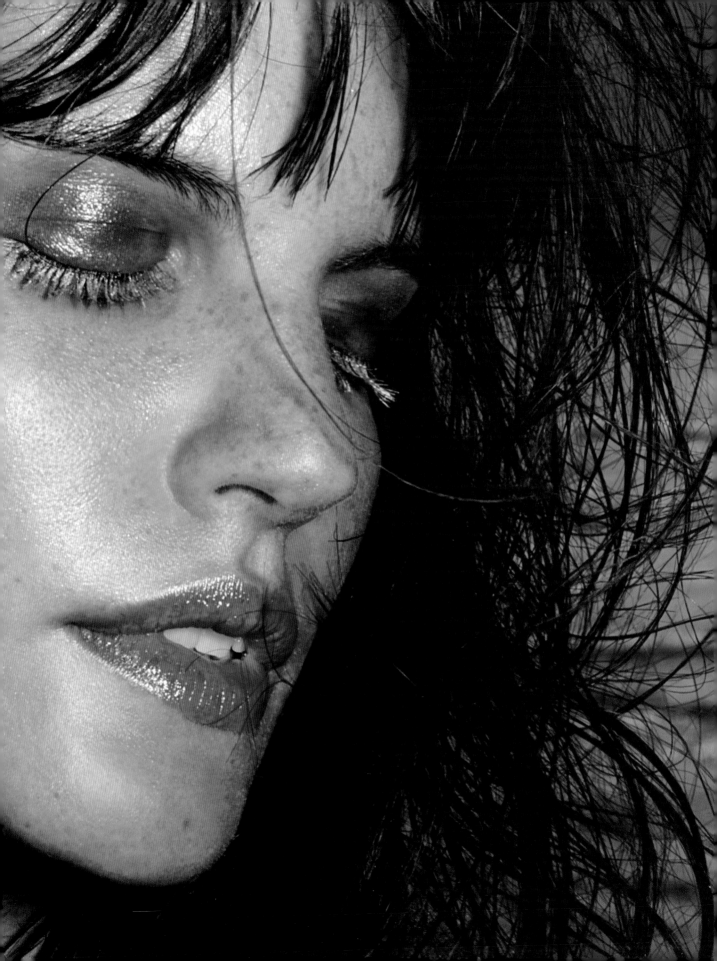

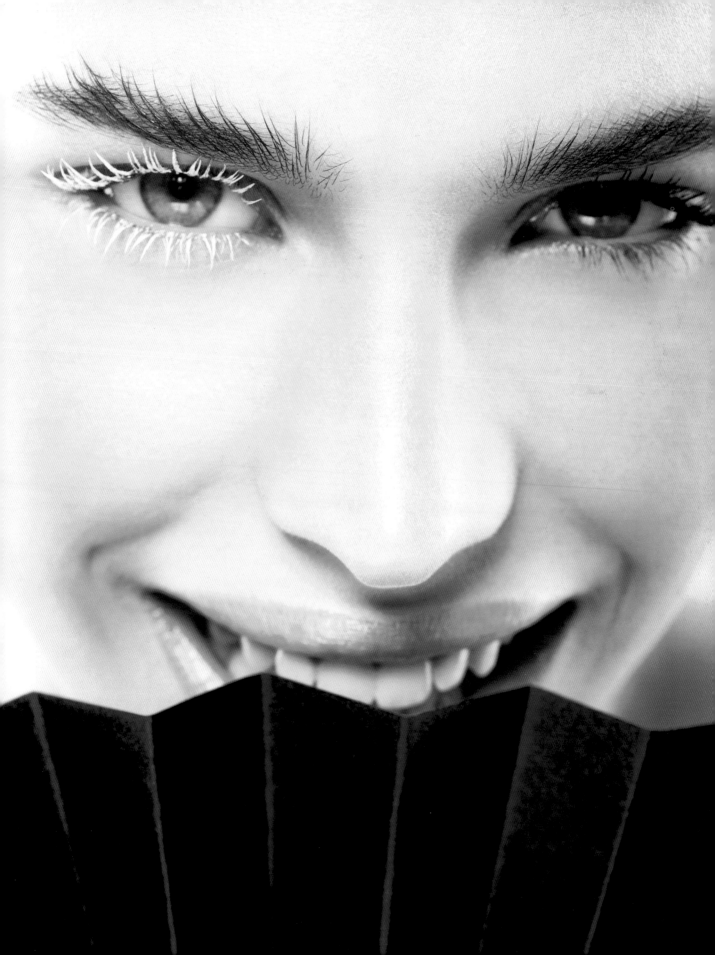

In the blink of an eye

Thickened, lengthened, or curled to perfection, maximize volume for the most glamorous lashes imaginable. Mascara sets the stage for an eye-stopping show.

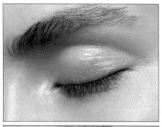

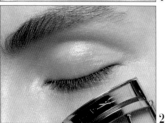

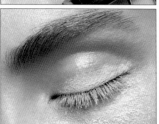

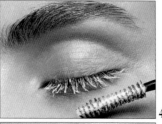

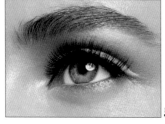

1 Your lashes should be **SPOTLESSLY CLEAN** before getting underway. Soothe your lids with a touch of concealer.

2 **LONG LIVE EYELASH CURLERS!** They are the preferred choice of professional makeup artists. But only use them on clean lashes otherwise you risk damaging or breaking them.

3 Here's one way to **THICKEN EYELASHES** before applying mascara: a (very light) veil of translucent powder.

4 If your mascara is a two-step process, start with a **LASH FORTIFIER** made from cellulose fibers that lengthens and thickens while it treats your lashes.

5 Apply mascara on the top of your lashes first, then from the roots, maintaining the curve in your movement. **FOR MAXIMUM VOLUME** leave the brush on the tips of freshly curled lashes for a few seconds. Start from the roots to ensure straight lashes instead of outward-pointing ones. Repeat the process until you have achieved the desired look.

ADVICE FROM IRÈNE OBERRAUCH (Studio makeup artist)
Make sure you close your mascara tightly so that it doesn't dry out. Contrary to popular belief, dipping the wand in and out does not ensure even distribution but instead dries out the product by forcing air into the tube.

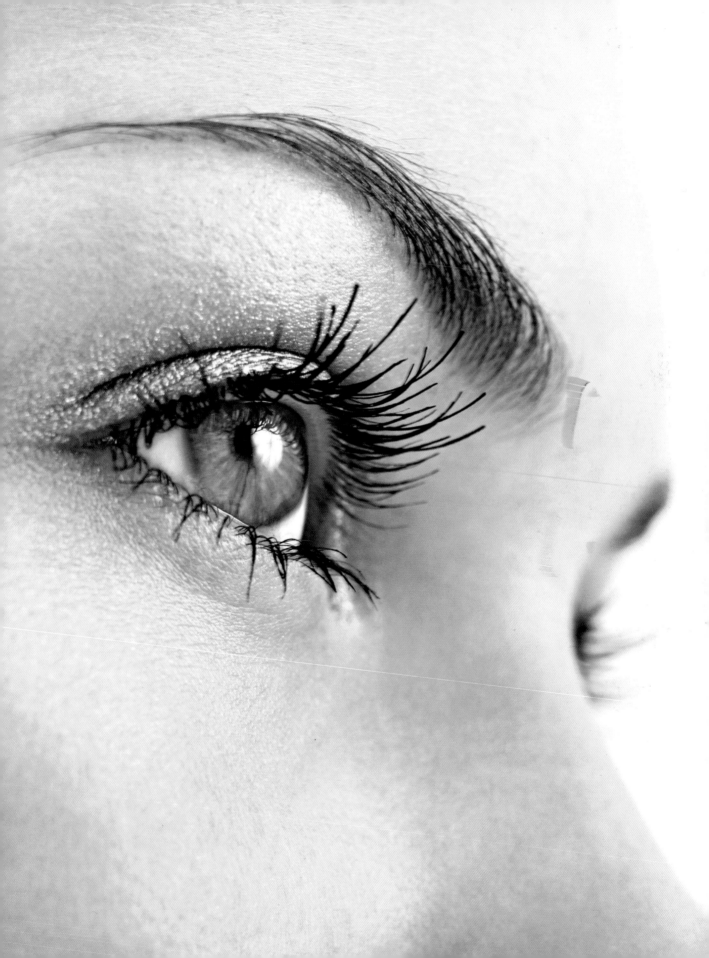

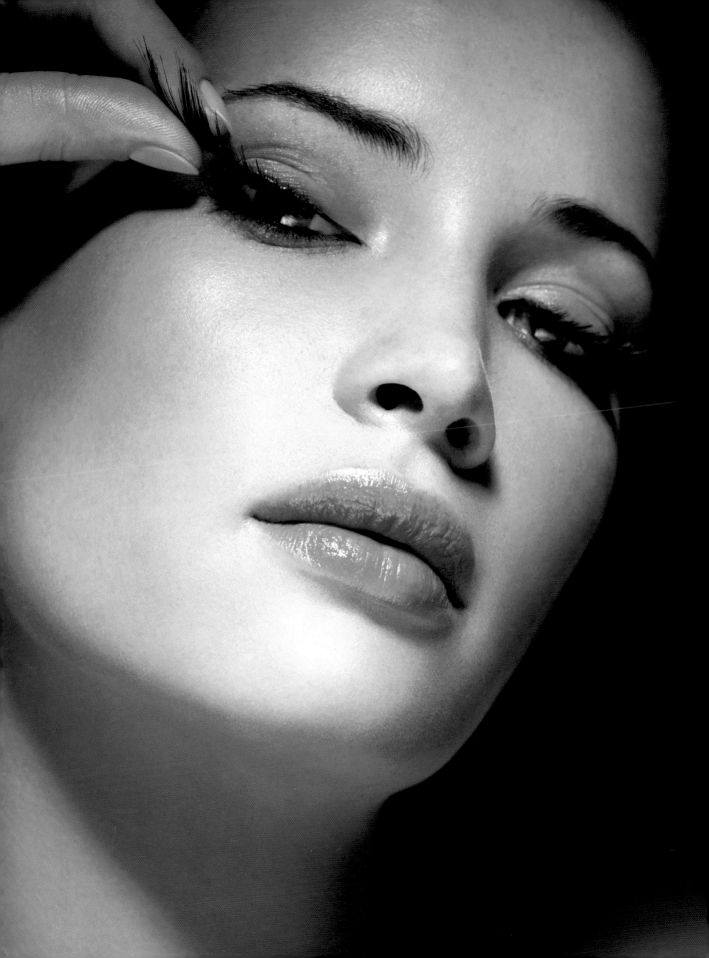

Fake is beautiful!

Make a short story long! Fake lashes go to great lengths to appear natural.

1 To get an idea of the final result, simply place the **FAKE LASHES** on top of your own: if you think they're too long, don't be afraid to trim them with scissors. Keep your hand steady and cut with one snip to guarantee a pretty shape.

2 **APPLY A THIN LINE** of eyelash glue to the base end of the fake lashes (with a little more on the edges since they're more likely to come loose). Blowing on the glue for a few seconds will ensure a better hold.

3 Starting from the inner corner, **PLACE THE LASHES** as close to your own lash line as possible.

4 While waiting for the glue to dry, gently **TAP THE LASHES** with the end of a brush for perfect positioning. Do your best not to blink so that the glue dries correctly.

5 **ROUND OFF THE LOOK** with a very thin line of eyeliner to blur the line where fake meets real. Mascara will guarantee as natural a look as possible.

ADVICE FROM LOUISE WITTLICH (Studio makeup artist)
Take your time. Finish one eye before starting the second.

How to remove them
Unstick them carefully, starting at the outer edge. Any remaining glue can easily be removed with sweet almond oil.

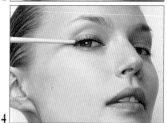

1

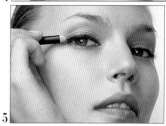

2

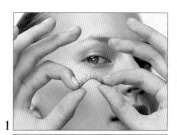

3

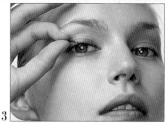

4

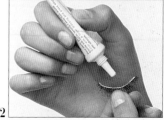

5

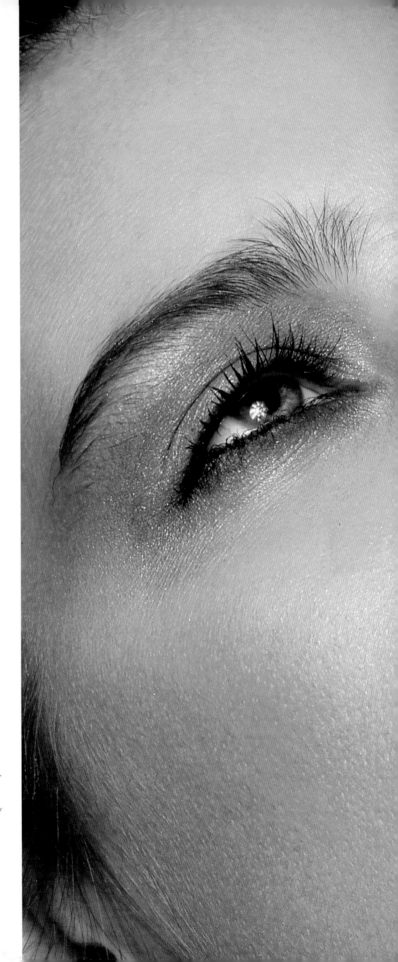

Powders
and
shadows
Perfectly
blended
For a
vibrant
canvas

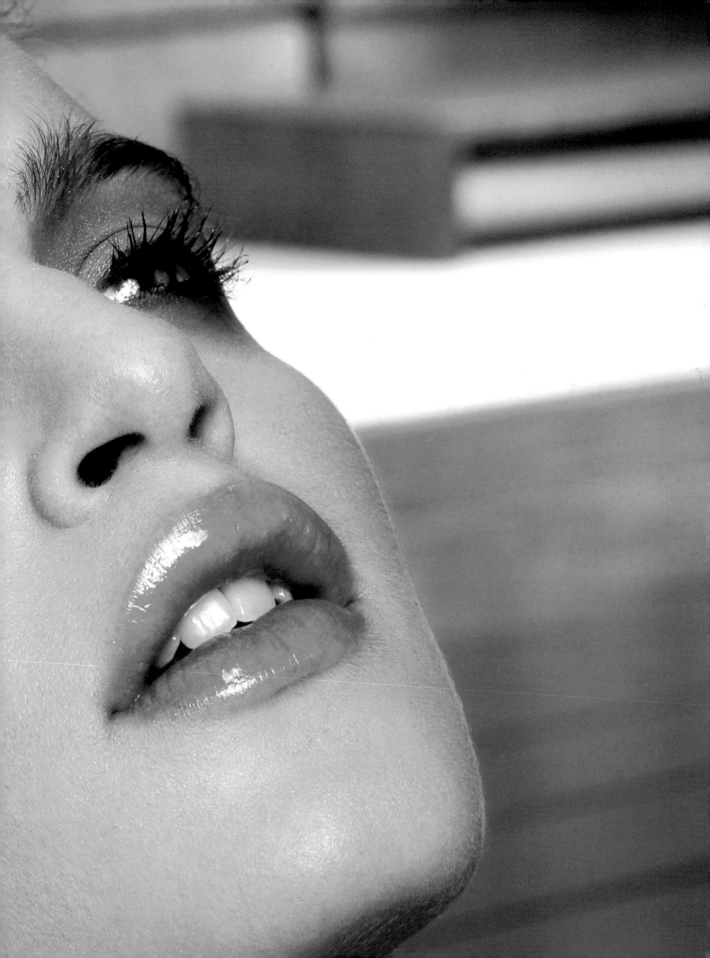

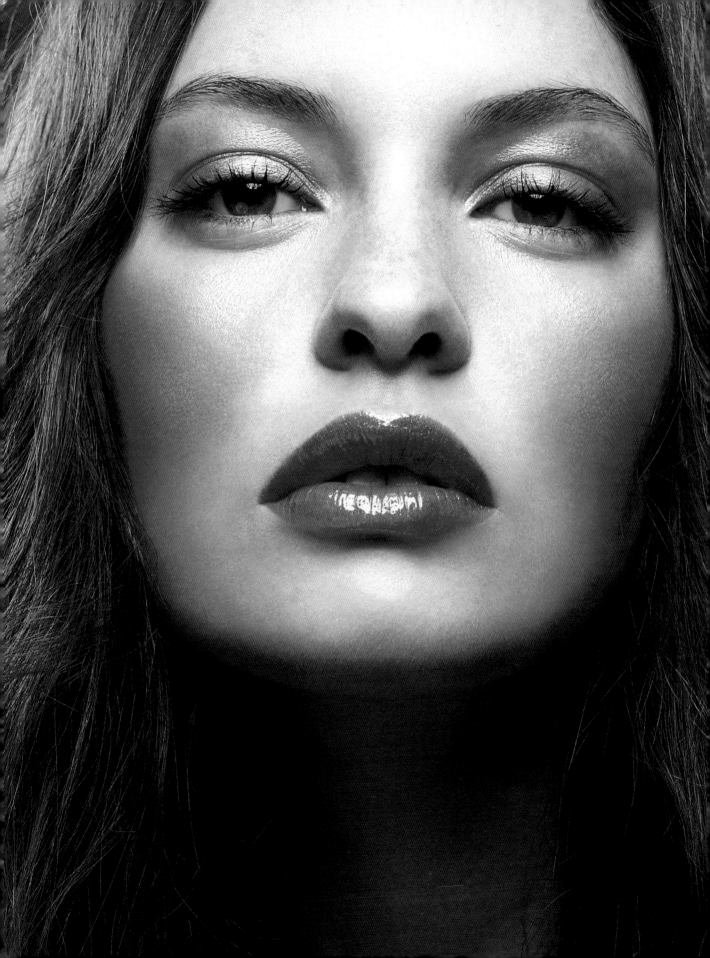

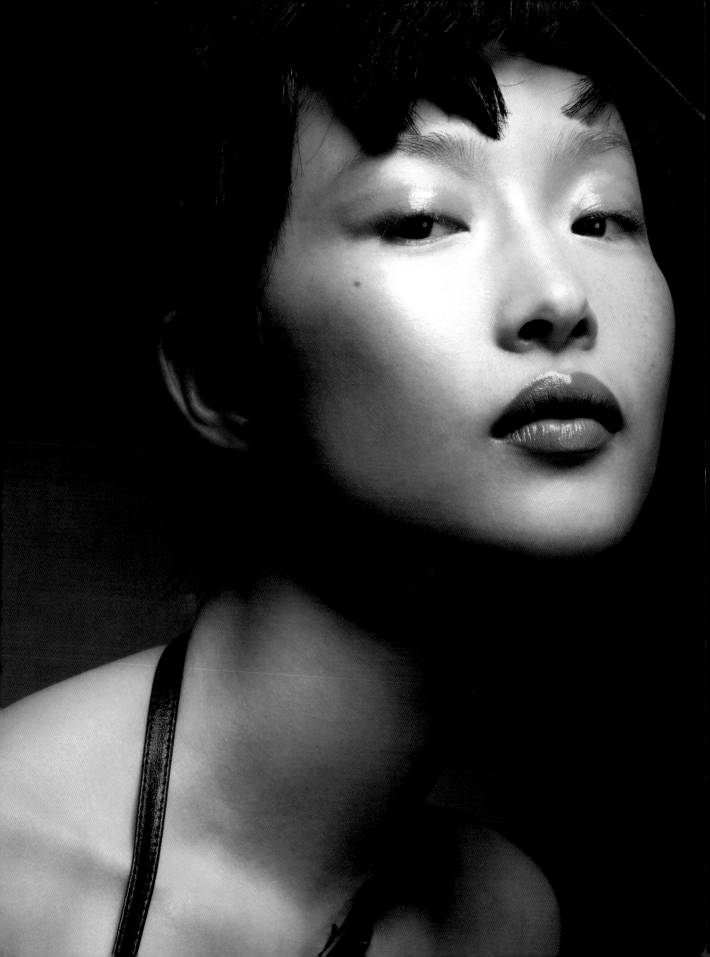

Where there's smoke, there's fire

It's a paradox: "smoky" tones bring light to your look.
With a skilled hand, plums become the new apple of your eye!

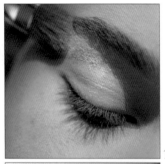

1

2

1 TO WIDEN YOUR EYES, use a lighter shade in the inner corner and fan outward with a darker one. If you're going for transparency, a brush is your best bet.

2 FOR A MORE INTENSE LOOK, just like on the outer edge of the eyelid shown here, use a dampened sponge brush dipped in shadow to blend for longer wear and more intense color.

Bigger A small touch of iridescent powder on the corner of your eyelids will make them look larger, so will a lighter shade dusted on your brow bones just under the eyebrows.

Deeper Running slightly over the outside edges will make them look less narrow. A halo effect around the arch (see photo at right) will also give depth.

A line of plum kohl pencil is a perfect finish for an elegant evening look.

ADVICE FROM SUZANNE STERLING (Chanel)
I recommend a flat, square-tipped brush for eyeshadow application. You can smudge with a rounded brush afterward. To magnify your eyes: put a small touch of a brighter powder smack in the middle of the upper lid.

What you'll need
- square brush
- round brush
- plum-colored eyeshadow
- light iridescent eyeshadow

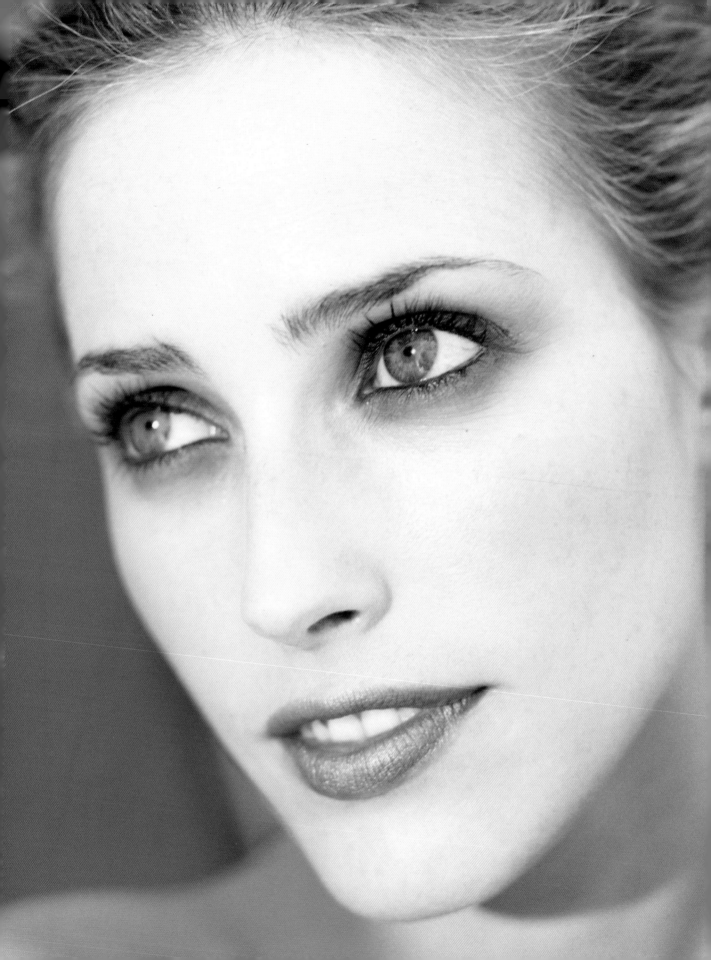

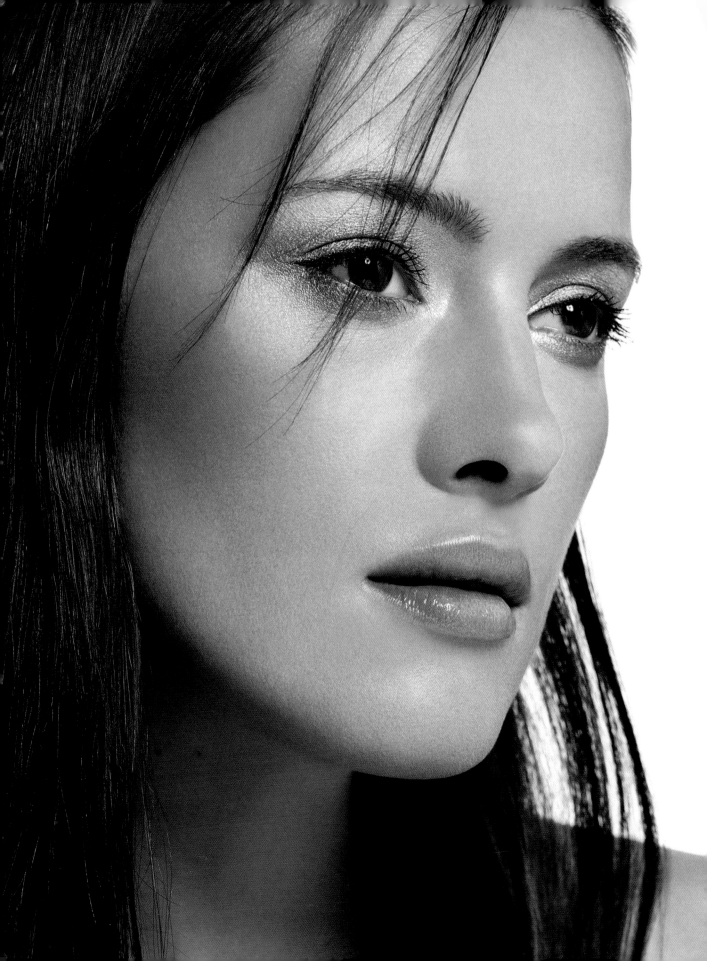

Metallic magic

Golden drops and silver powders are refined but not too flashy. Let the party begin!

1 Again, use **EYELASH CURLERS** only on clean lashes and start at the roots. Curlers will prevent you from overdoing it with mascara.

2 Blend in **CONCEALER** under your eye, from the inner to outer corners, following the lash line.

3 **USE A BRUSH** to apply the first coppery coat at the base of your eyelid, starting from the inside corner and then under your lower lashes. Add a silvery note and blend upward toward your eyebrows.

4 **SKETCH** a pearly V on the inner corner of your eye to give a touch of light.

5 Keeping your eyelid taut, **DRAW A THIN LINE** of eyeliner from the inside, working your way out, and finish off with a coat of mascara.

ADVICE FROM JAMES KALIARDOS (L'Oréal Paris)
Opt for a kohl pencil if you are tired of liquid eyeliner.

What you'll need
- eyelash curler
- narrow brush
- thick eyeshadow brush
- concealer
- copper shadow
- silver shadow eyeliner

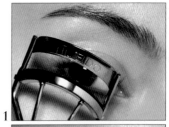
1

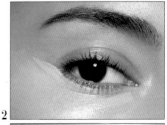
2

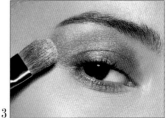
3

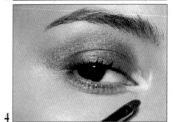
4

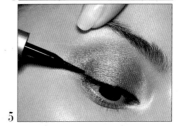
5

.Iridescent irises

Pink diamond and plum pearl: an irresistible pairing that will light up any pair of eyes

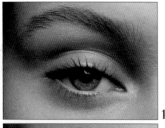

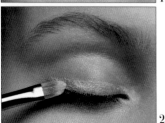

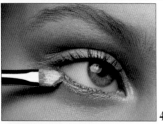

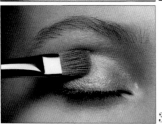

1 With your eyebrows flawlessly brushed and your lashes curled with the help of your eyelash curler, **LEAVE YOUR LID BARE:** cream eyeshadow will stay perfectly in place.

2 With your eye closed, **PLACE THE CREAMY PINK SHADOW** on the lid, spreading and blending from the lash line with a flat brush.

3 Using a larger, clean brush, **BLEND UPWARD** toward your brow bone to achieve total transparency.

4 While looking up, **DRAW A LINE** of plum shadow under your eye, working out from the inner corner.

5 For an even more sophisticated effect, **SMUDGE A BIT** with your finger, in the direction of your temple, before putting on mascara.

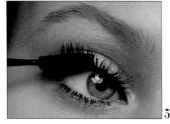

ADVICE FROM JULIE NOZIERS (Studio makeup artist)
If the result is too sparkly, use some translucent powder to tone it down. And for perfect hold, only apply powder around your eyes after you have completely finished putting on your makeup.

What you'll need

- eyelash curler
- small and narrow eyeshadow brush
- full eyeshadow brush
- pink cream eyeshadow
- plum cream eyeshadow

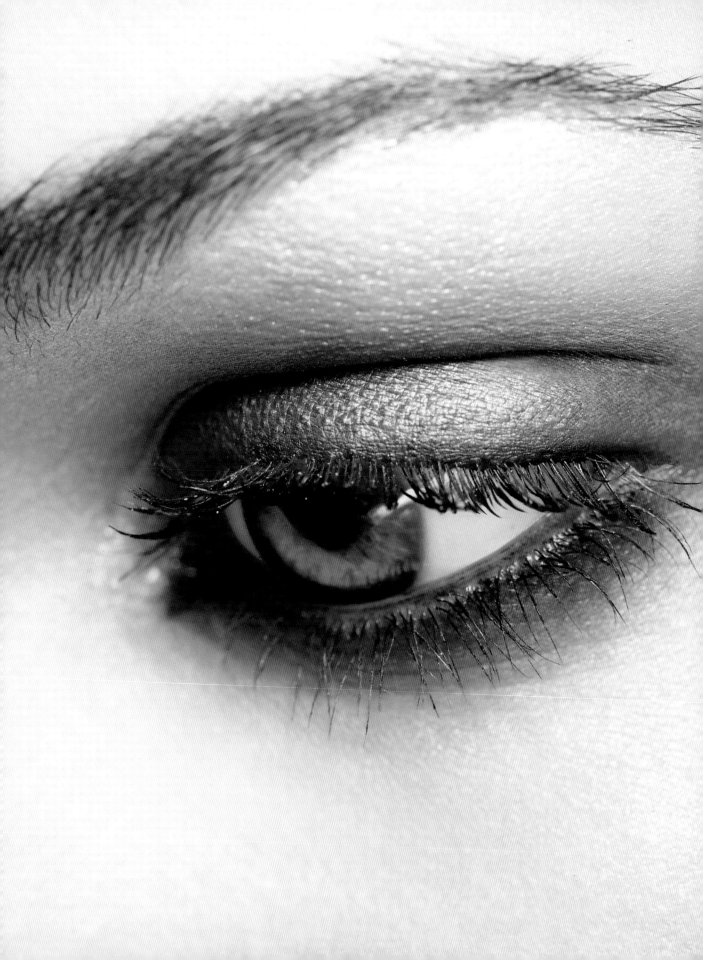

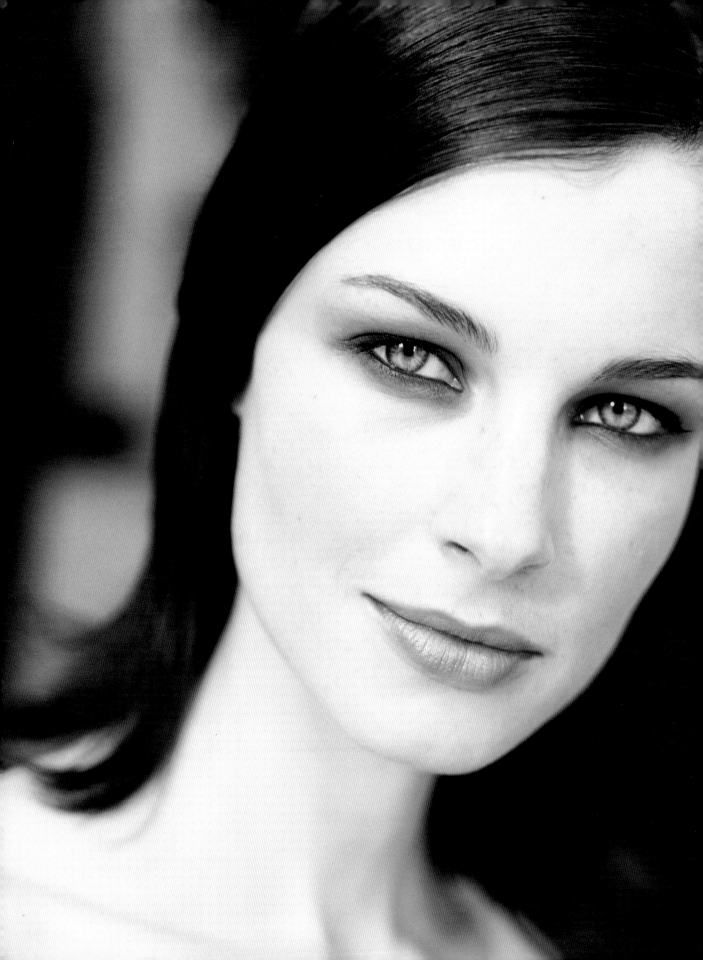

Velvety sweetness

A powdery setting for your eyes will bring out the light in your gaze and give it depth and mystery. A velvety matte gray will do the trick.

APPLIED WITH YOUR FINGERS, smoky shades of creamy eyeshadow will yield magnificent color gradation.

They adapt to your desired intensity instantly during the day … or night! Microscopic pigments give rise to flattering colors that are both **intense and transparent.** You can apply a darker tone on the entire eyelid and then blend before overlaying a lighter shade.

FOR EVENINGS, you can bring the color up to your brow bones, highlighting and creating a halo effect mirrored under your eyes.

For this look, go easy on the mascara: opt for length rather than volume.

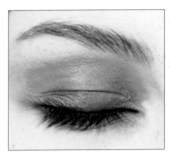

Gradation creates a soft, blurred effect over the whole lid that brightens up the under-eyebrow arch.

ADVICE FROM OLIVIER ÉCHAUDEMAISON (Guerlain)
An elegant alternative to black, which can end up too harsh, smoky grays give you a refined look that intensifies dark eyes and adds clarity and depth to lighter eyes.

What you'll need
- smoky gray cream eyeshadow
- lengthening mascara

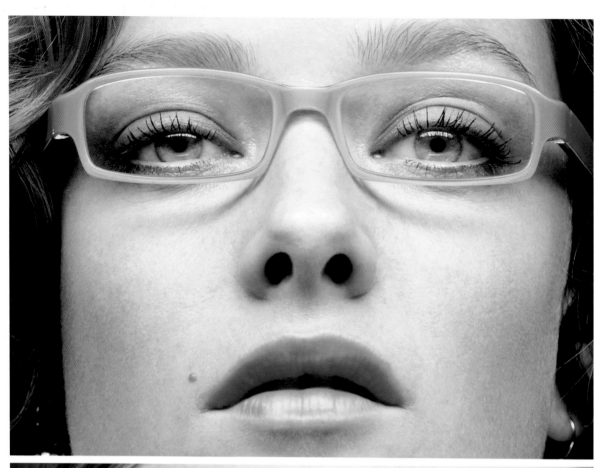

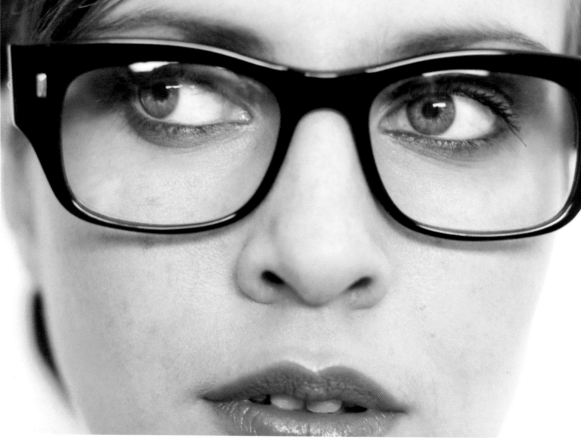

Focus on glasses

Maintain the intensity of your gaze under the lens.

Regardless of the shape of your glasses, **OPT FOR FULLY TREATED GLASS LENSES.** Choose an anti-reflective coating for your lenses that will keep the splendor of your eyes intact. With an untreated lens all your makeup efforts will be wasted!

IF YOU ARE NEARSIGHTED, your glasses might have a tendency to make your eyes look smaller. Reinforce your features with eyeliner and use extra mascara as well.

IF YOU ARE FARSIGHTED, your eyes will look larger through your glasses. Definitely flattering, but the magnifying effect is ruthless. James Kaliardos recommends taking great care in choosing brushes and mascara in order to have well-separated eyelashes and prevent any unattractive build-up. For the same reason, eyeshadow must also be blended with great care.

ADVICE FROM JAMES KALIARDOS (L'Oréal Paris) Choose your brushes according to how you plan on using them and clean them regularly, especially since your eyes are far more sensitive and prone to allergies than other areas of your face.

Touch-up work: To make up for mistakes in eyeliner or mascara application, erase the slip-up with a cotton swab dipped in concealer. Next, dip the same swab in loose powder and apply to the area that needs to be redone.

You're the star of the show, Pretty as a picture.

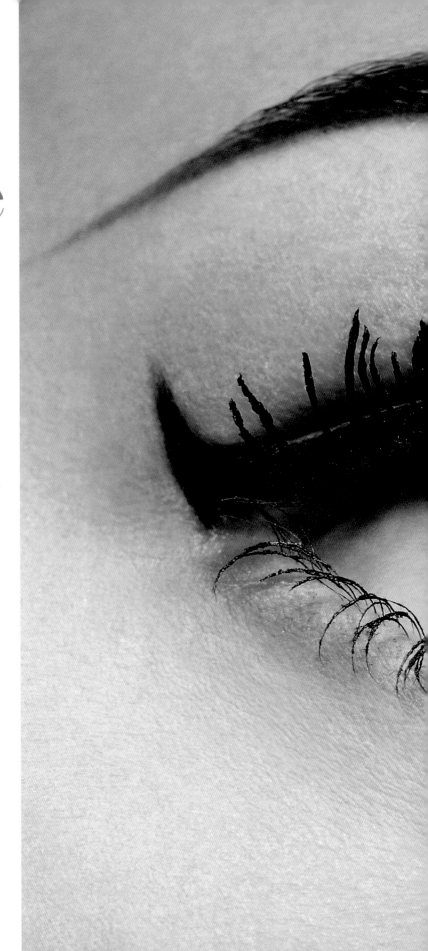

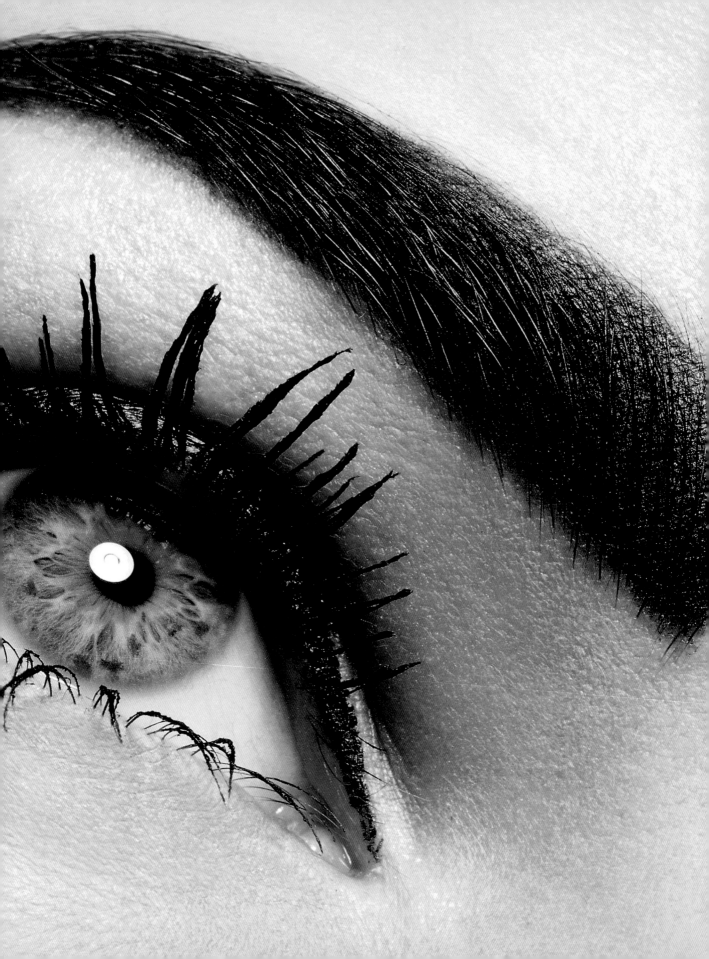

Staying in shape

*Straight, arched, comma-shaped, or like an arrow. . .
the shape of your eyebrows is a defining factor of your look.*

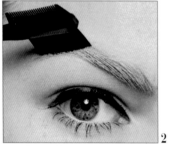

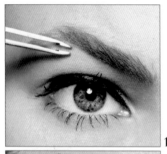

1 BEFORE TWEEZING, comb your eyebrows in the opposite direction of growth and then straighten them by combing the other way. Pull your skin taut using your thumb and index finger, and tweeze in direction of growth. Don't overdo it: only pluck eyebrows on the underside, and thin out the brow as you work outward. The middle should remain thick. Keep an eye on your brows (as hair grows back quickly) in order to keep the arch clearly defined with occasional touch-ups.

TECHNIQUES FOR A BALANCED FACE

For close-set eyes Maintain full brows from the inner corner of your eye to the arch.

To look younger Keep your brows short with a shape that stops before the edge of your eye. A well-defined eyebrow shape gives energy to your expression. Raising the line energizes your face.

2 Once you've combed your eyebrows into place, your brow pencil, chosen in the same shade as your eyebrows (or one shade lighter, but never darker!) will help you **THICKEN AND CORRECT** minor tweezing errors by using short, thin lines drawn in the direction of growth. Always use upward movements and work outward from the inner corner of your eye. Blend it all together with a cotton swab.

ADVICE FROM NICOLAS DEGENNES (Givenchy)
I would suggest using a pencil rather than a shadow—which results in too "harsh" of a look—to highlight the top of your eyebrows, never the underside.

The right length
Eyebrows should run from the inner to the outer corners of your eyes. It may be wise to start off with professional brow shaping and then keep up the form with occasional plucking at home.

What you'll need
- tweezers
- eyebrow comb
- sharp-tipped eyebrow pencil

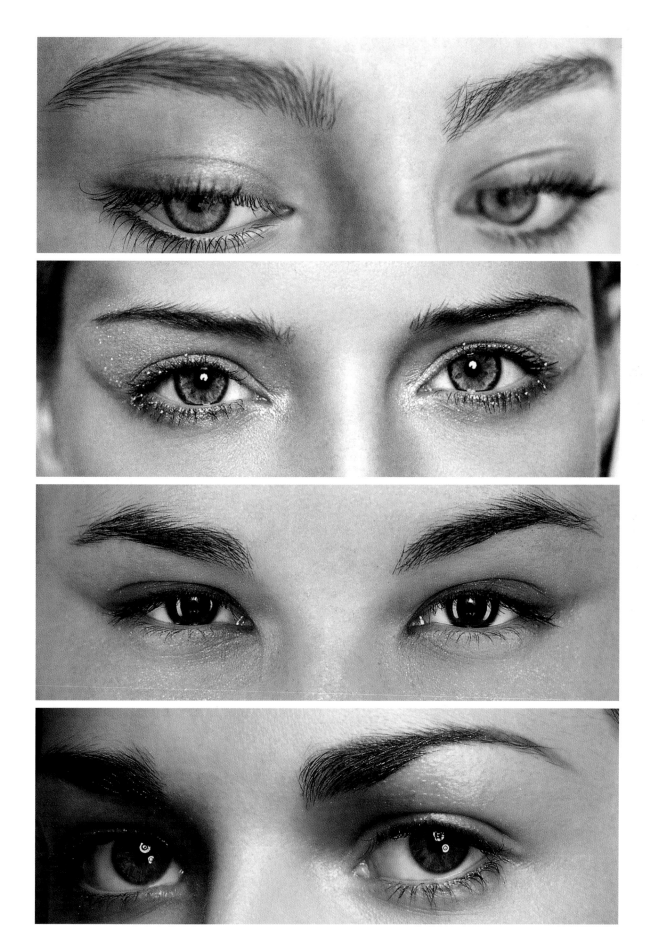

Brooke or Audrey...
Starry eyes

It's amazing how a little doting on your eyebrows can totally transform your look.

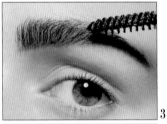
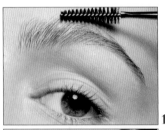
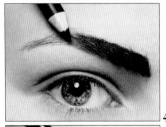
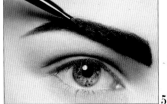

FOR A BROOKE SHIELDS LOOK (TOM PECHEUX, SHISEIDO)

1 Your brows should be **straightened by upward combing,** without breaking the line, in order to give an impression of greater width.

2 **Fill in with a pencil** (black to dark brown for dark-haired women; gray to light brown for blondes) using short, feathery strokes, starting along the underside.

3 **Blend in using an eyebrow wand,** then with a coat of clear mascara to maximize volume.

FOR AN AUDREY HEPBURN LOOK (TERRY, BY TERRY)

4 For an intensely sculpted brow: **fill in eyebrows with a pencil** in a robust shade that goes with your hair, working outward from your nose.

5 **Even out with a brush,** while drawing a well-groomed line tapering elegantly at the ends. The brush will fill in the natural shape of your eyebrows while distributing color. Use dry beauty oil or clear mascara for the final touch.

What you'll need
- professional eyebrow tweezers
- eyebrow comb
- beveled-edge eyebrow brush
- eyebrow wand
- eyebrow pencil
- clear eyebrow mascara

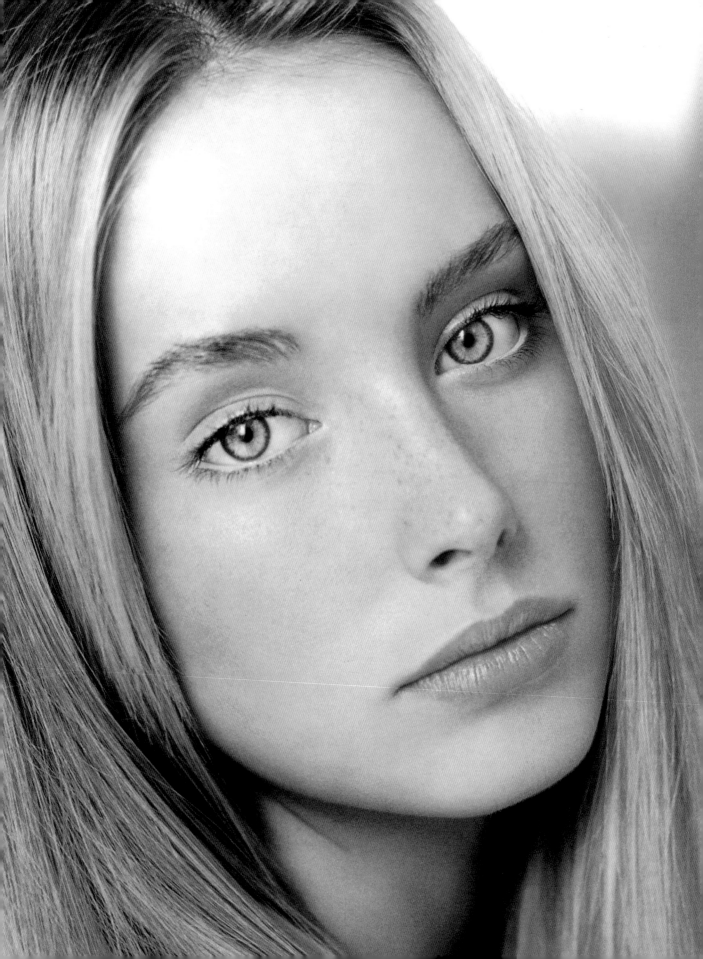

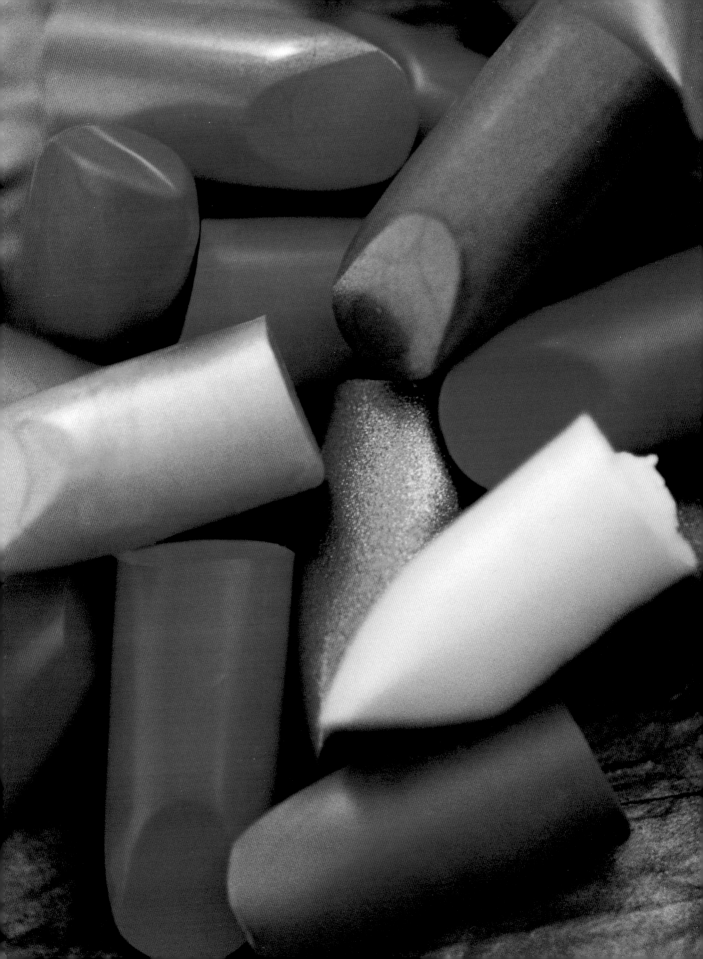

4Lips

WORD OF MOUTH

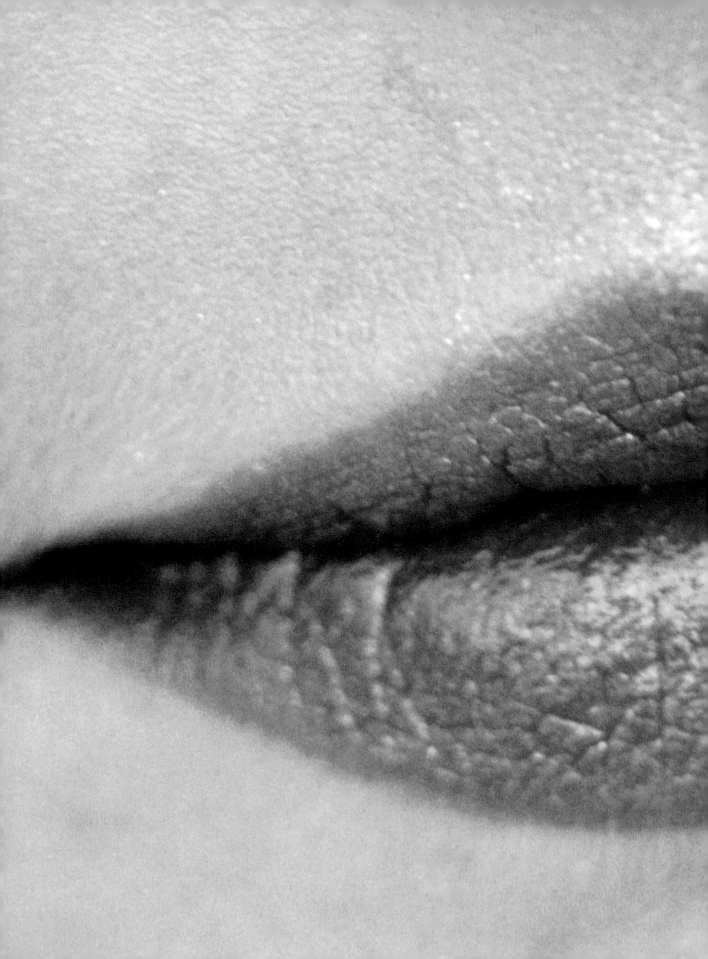

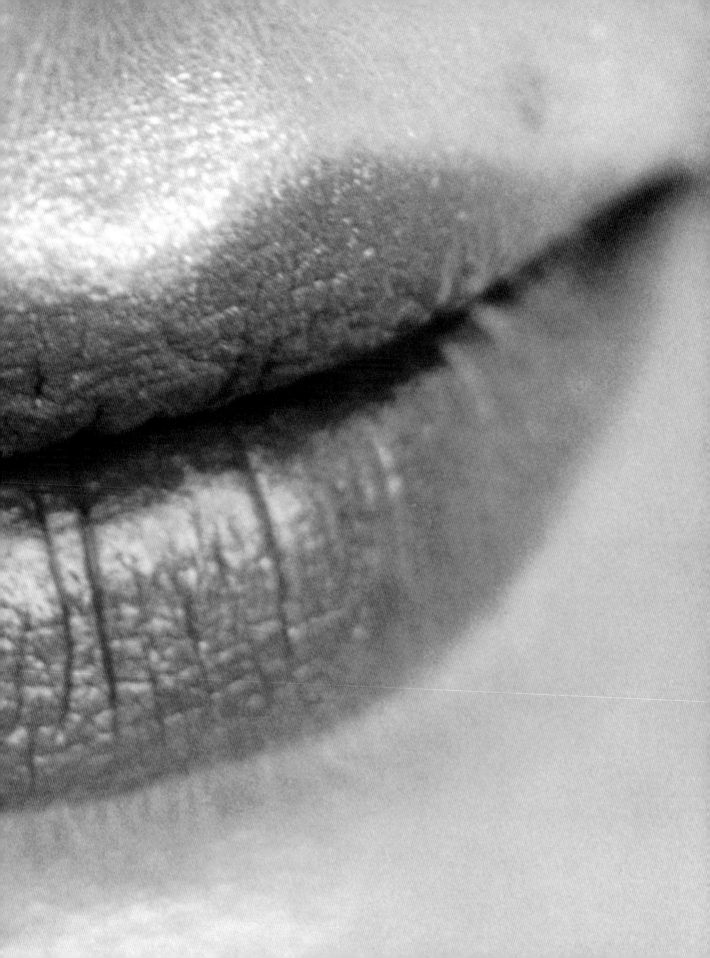

Fresh and natural perfectly pink

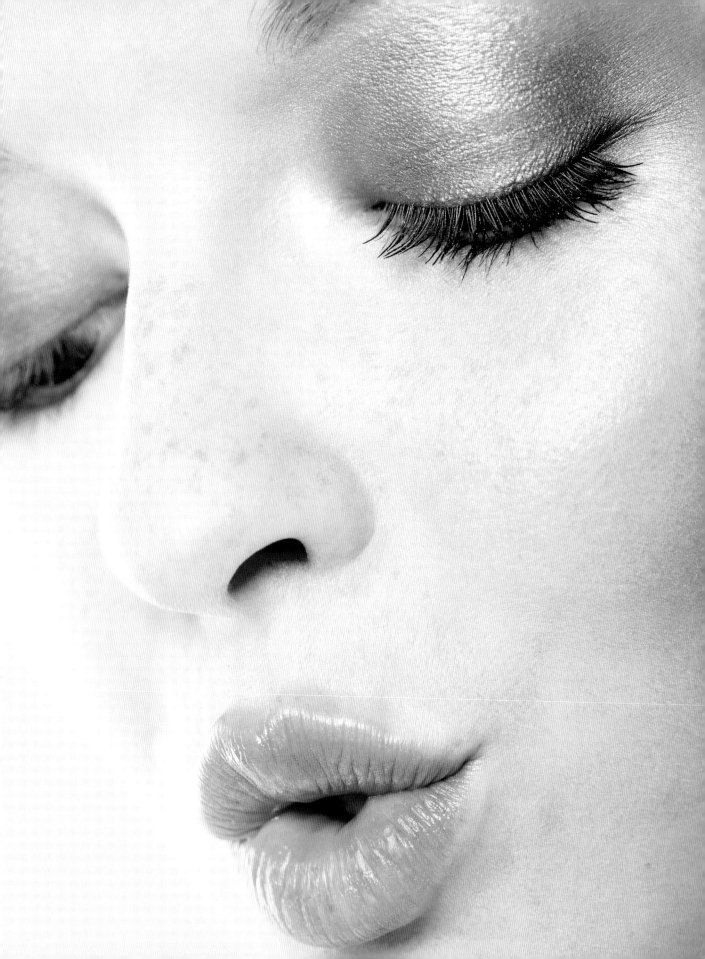

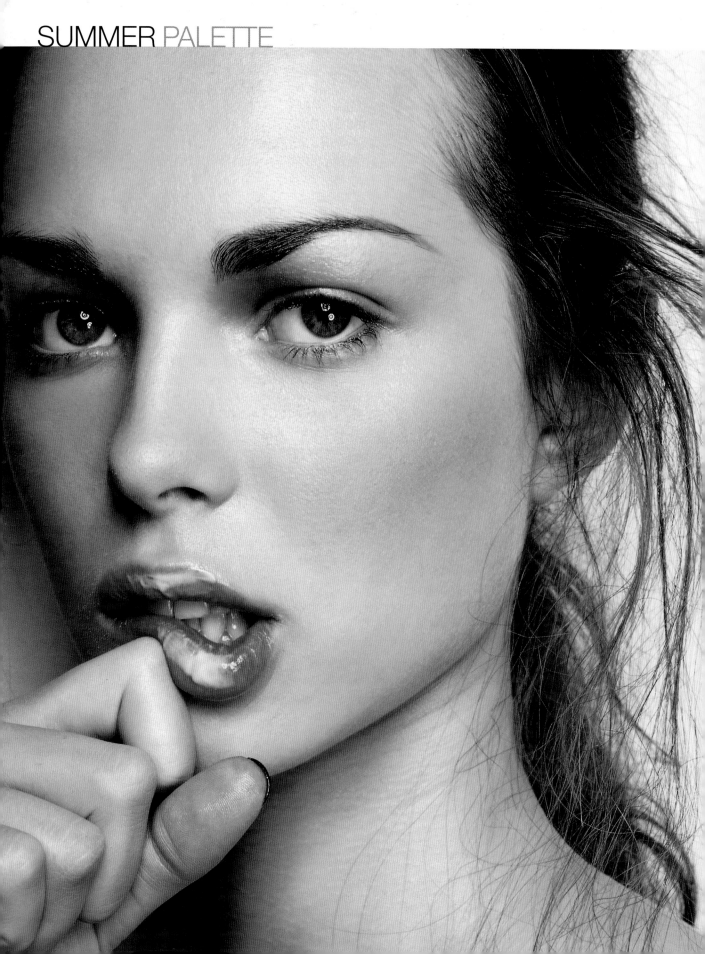

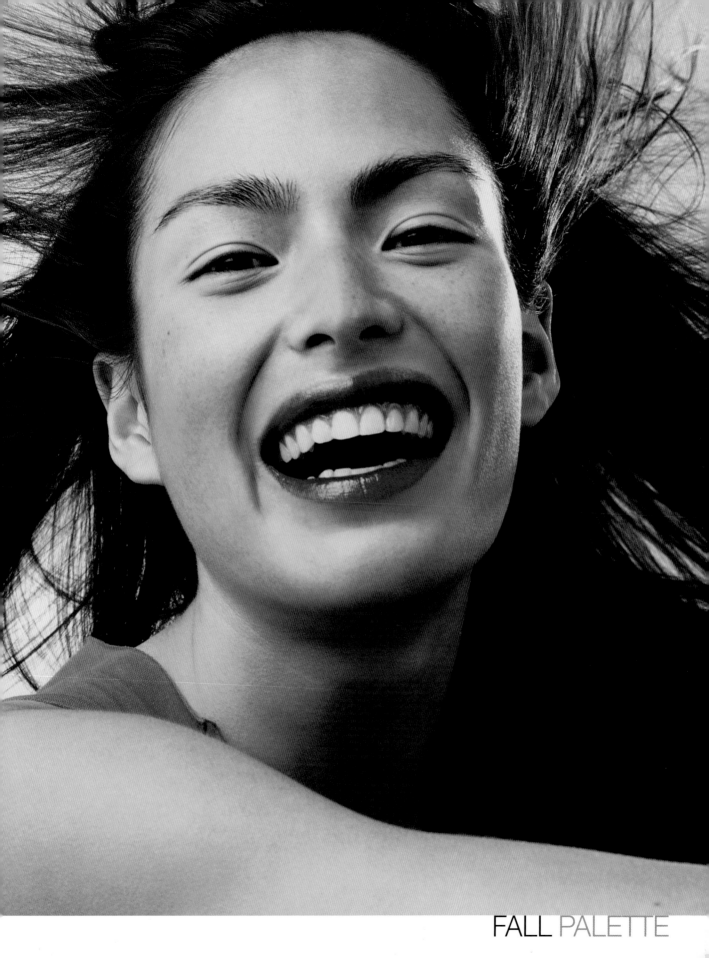

FALL PALETTE

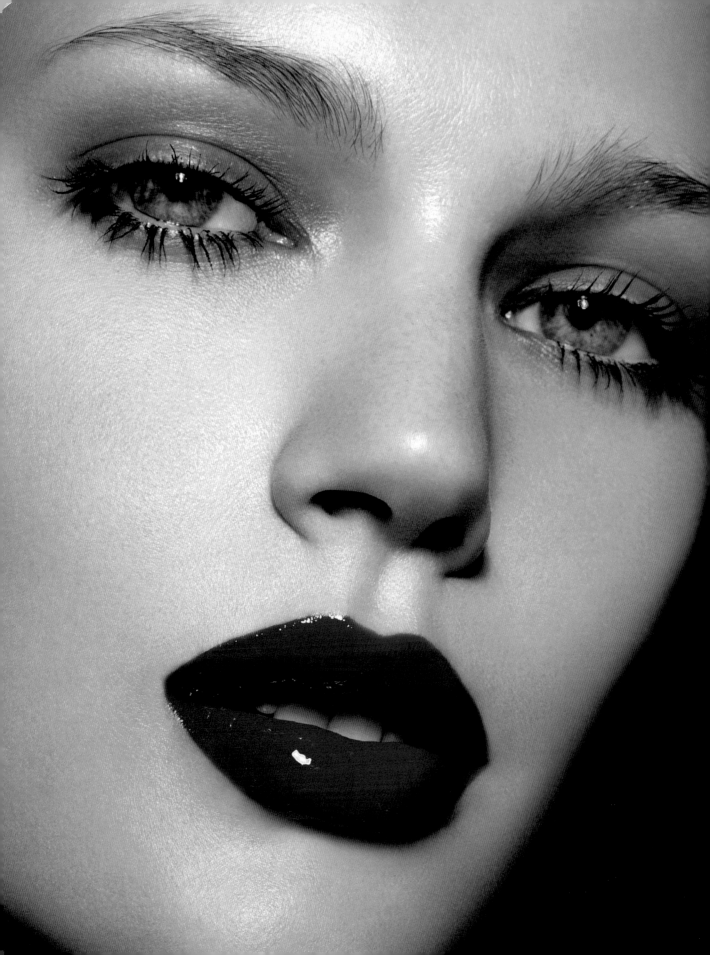

High
beams
red lights—
Full
speed
ahead

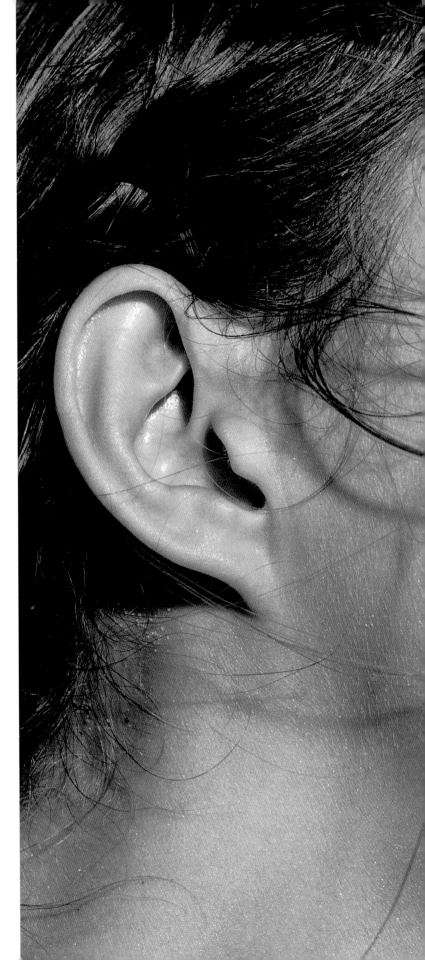

Exquisite
Sweet
as candy
Good
enough to
eat

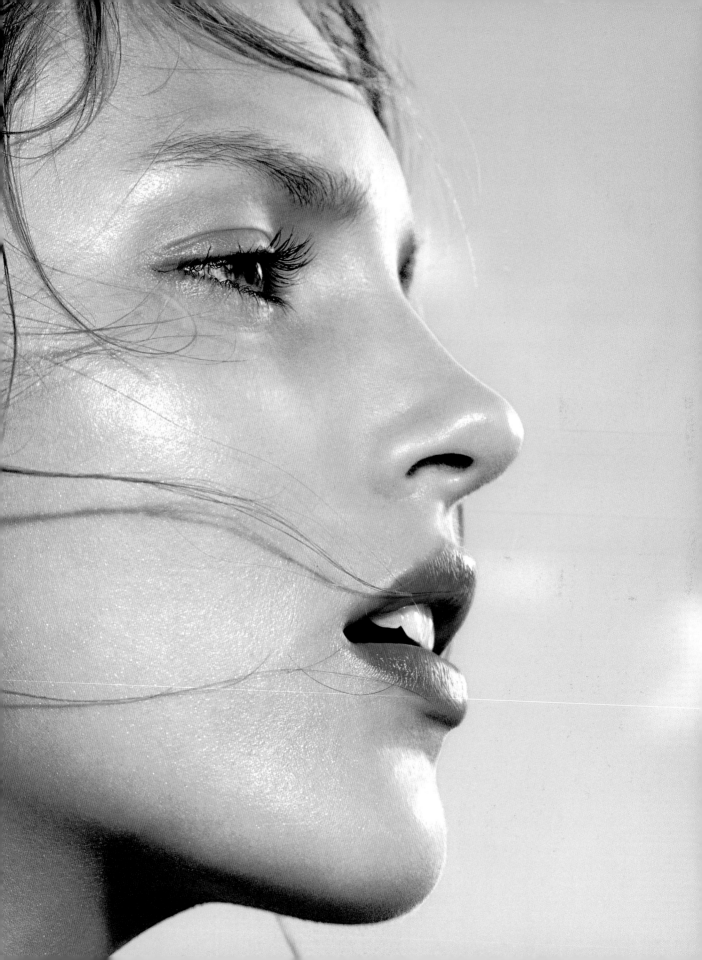

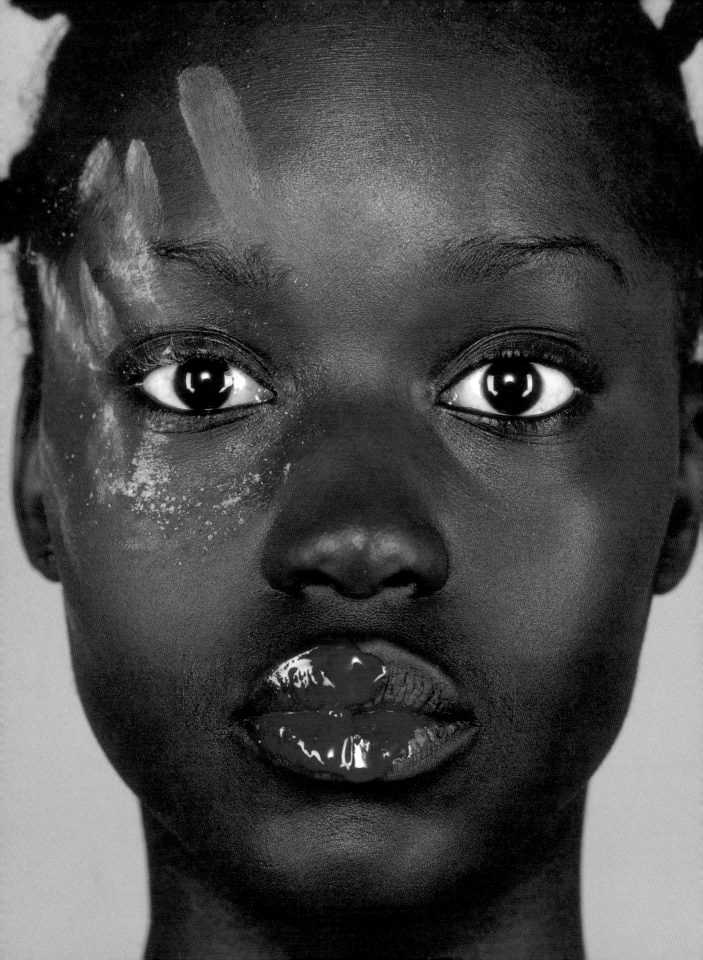

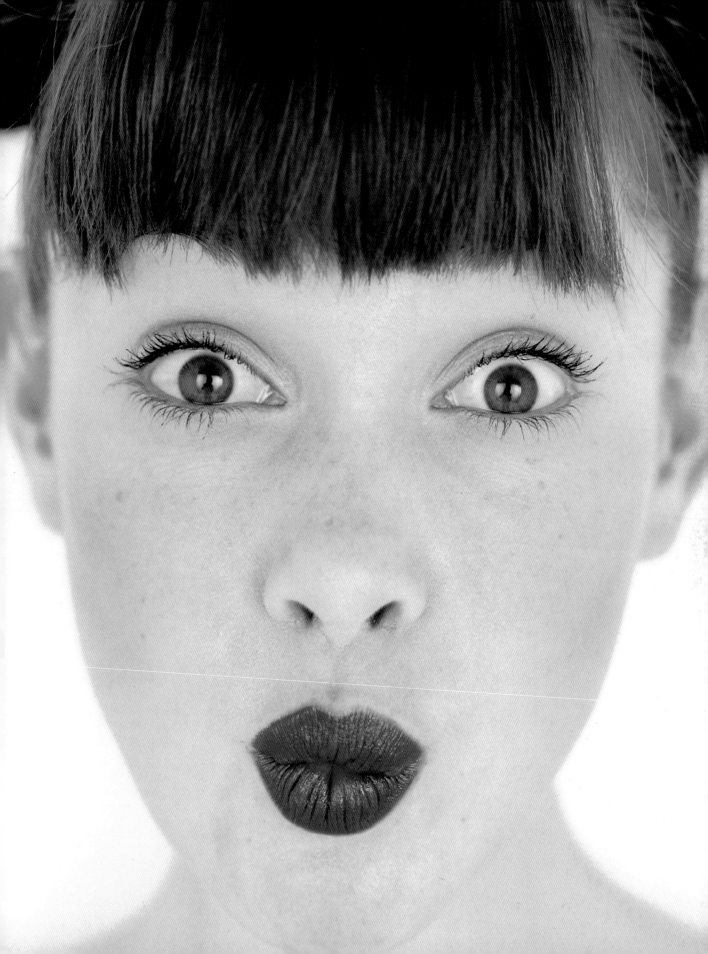

Fire-engine red or sensual nude?

What's important in choosing a lipstick? Your complexion, the color of your eyes and hair, the shape of your mouth? Down with preconceptions. Let's hear it for making yourself feel good, in every color!

Don't believe everything you're told! A bold red can be sublime on a blonde, just like beige can be gorgeous on a brunette.

WE AREN'T LIVING IN A MONOCHROME WORLD anymore (matching lips, blush, and eyeshadow). Aim for balance, however. If you're going to accentuate your lips, then compensate by going easy on your eyes.

SMALL MOUTHS are better off with a very light shade like beige (or "nude"). A color that's too dark tends to accentuate the thinness of your lips.

PLUMP LIPS call for darker shades that will paradoxically draw attention away from your mouth.

Don't be afraid of bold colors! It's up to you. The glossier your lipstick, the easier it will be to wear: matte lipsticks can make your face look harsh, while **ULTRA-FLATTERING GLOSSY SHADES** bring out the best in your lips. Deep red lipstick is a miracle worker: it will make your teeth appear whiter, has a blushing effect, and instantly gives you a sophisticated air.

ADVICE FROM NOLWENN DU LAZ (journalist at Marie Claire Paris)
Want to try a new color for that special evening? Test it during the day and see what reactions you receive. If you get the thumbs up, you're ready for a night out on the town!

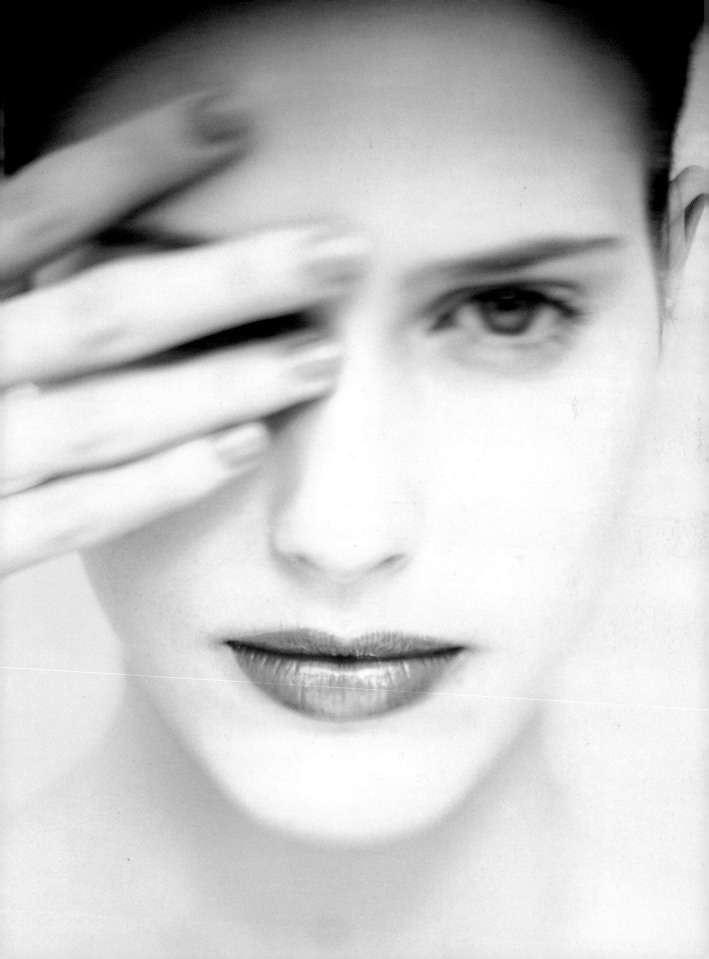

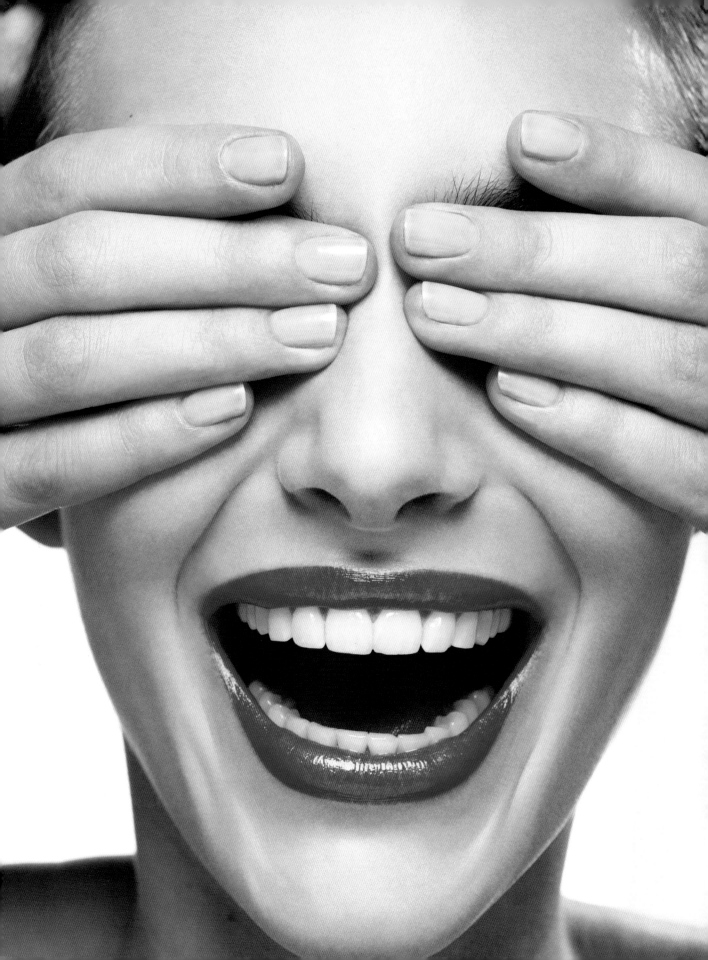

Fingers vs. pencils

Choose the right tools for application.
And don't forget your lip liner, a faithful fix-it-all.

1 For a natural, deliberately imperfect appearance that is soft and muted, apply lipstick to the flat of your index finger and **DELICATELY DAB ON COLOR** from one corner of your mouth to the other—without forgetting the interior of the lip—for an irresistible "just kissed" look.

2 **LIP PENCILS** are not only for lining the lip: they also help prevent your lipstick from bleeding and collecting in the small wrinkles around your mouth. They will also help you achieve a more matte look.

TIPS FOR A PERFECT POUT

To correct: **droopy lips** Try a touch of concealer around both corners of your mouth before lining your lips with a pencil, moving along toward your upper lip. **small lips** (photo 3) Try a thin line of beige lip pencil just beyond the natural lines of your mouth, thinning toward the inside of your lips in order to go past your natural lip line with color… stick with light colors and iridescent formulas. **full lips** (photo 4) Try a layer of foundation on the entire mouth, with a thin pencil line contouring your lips. Fill it in with similar tones using the lightest shade near the corners of your mouth. Avoid dark colors: with full lips, they attract attention but not necessarily in a good way.

ADVICE FROM TERRY (By TERRY) The multi-layered secret
After applying your lipstick, use a thick pencil to draw a series of vertical lines across your lips before applying a second coat of lipstick. Top it off with a final swipe of pencil to keep it all in place. You'll achieve excellent hold and the fantastic illusion of fuller lips.

What you'll need
- lipstick
- lip pencil

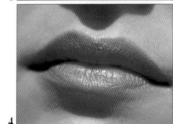

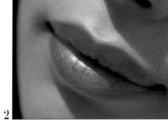

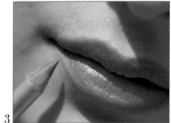

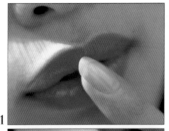

Red: A timeless classic

Immortalized by Coco Chanel and reinvented countless times, red lipstick remains the unquestionable mark of timeless elegance.

1 **VINTAGE REDS...IN STICKS** Applying lipstick is the epitome of sensuality and an act of irresistible femininity. With lipsticks coming in an unending variety of colors and textures, you can put your creativity and imagination to work.

2 **STICK TRICK** Apply color to the back of your hand first. This technique warms the product to ensure maximal hold. Then dab the desired amount onto lips.

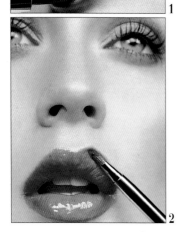

ADVICE FROM A PROFESSIONAL MAKEUP ARTIST (Stila)
The same lip brush will help you both accent the natural lines of your mouth and color the inside of your lips.

What you'll need
- lipstick
- thin and flat lip brush

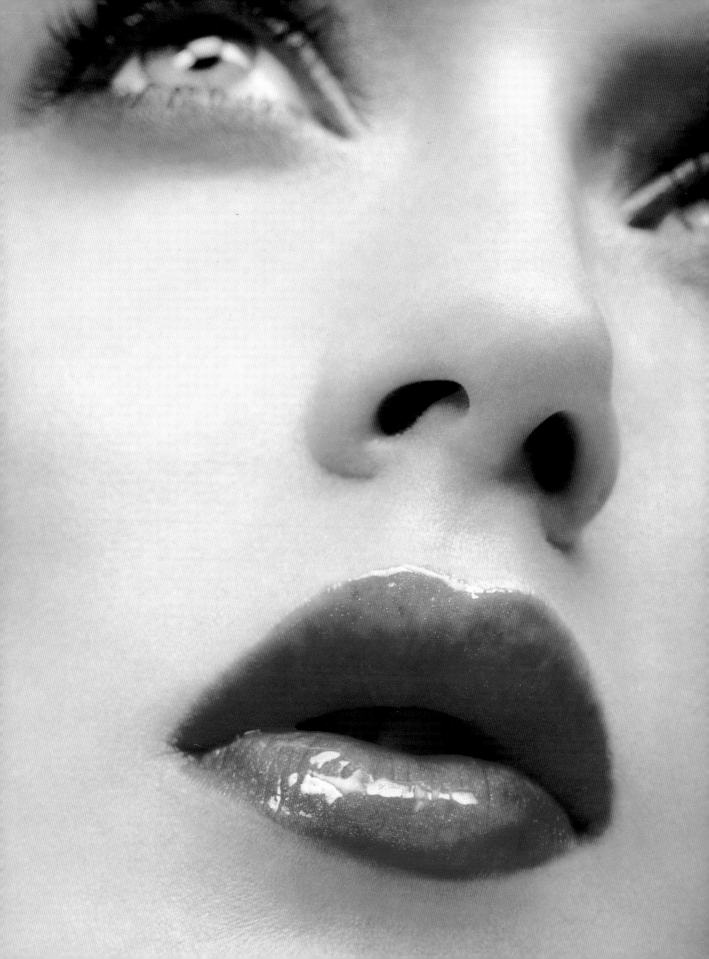

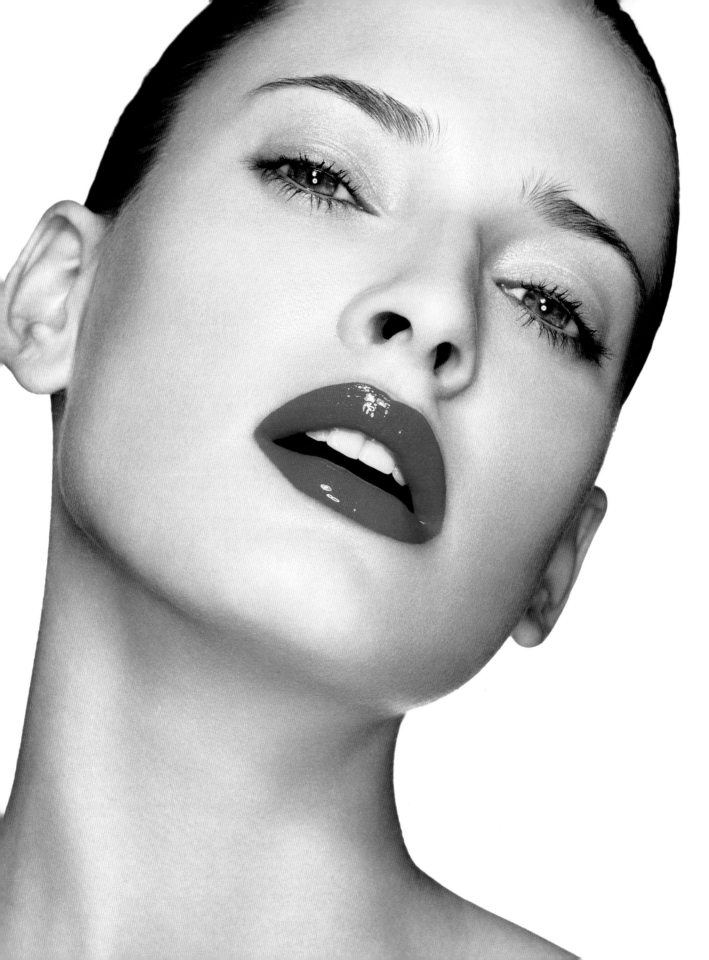

Secrets for luscious lips

Looking for lips as appetizing as juicy, fresh fruit? Here are five easy steps to follow for a perfect finish.

1 Like your skin, your mouth also needs to rid itself of dead cells from time to time. **FOR SILKY LIPS** choose a very soft facial exfoliant and gently clean away with a soft, supple toothbrush (reserved exclusively for this purpose).

2 Generously apply an **ULTRA-RICH, CREAMY LIP BALM** (or even Vaseline) for several minutes to nourish your lips. Wipe away with a cotton swab when done.

3 Think of your **LIP LINER** as your lips' guardrails. It should be the same color as your lipstick, but one shade lighter. Nude tones will suit paler complexions and will yield a flattering effect of increased volume.

4 Coat both sides of the brush with lipstick and start **APPLYING FROM THE INSIDE** of your lips, moving upward in small strokes until you reach the outer edges.

5 Lip gloss will help bring it all together: a single dollop in the middle of your lips will create a dynamic three-dimensional effect. Of course you can also spread it across your whole lip for a **FULL-ON SHINE.**

What you'll need
- soft-tipped lip pencil
- flat lip brush (no more than 1/5 inch)
- vibrant lipstick
- lip gloss, either clear or the same color as the lipstick

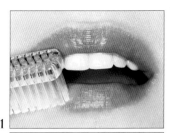

1

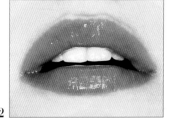

2

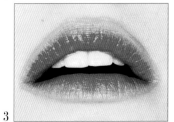

3

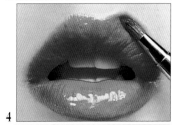

4

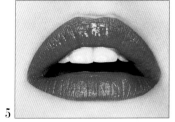

5

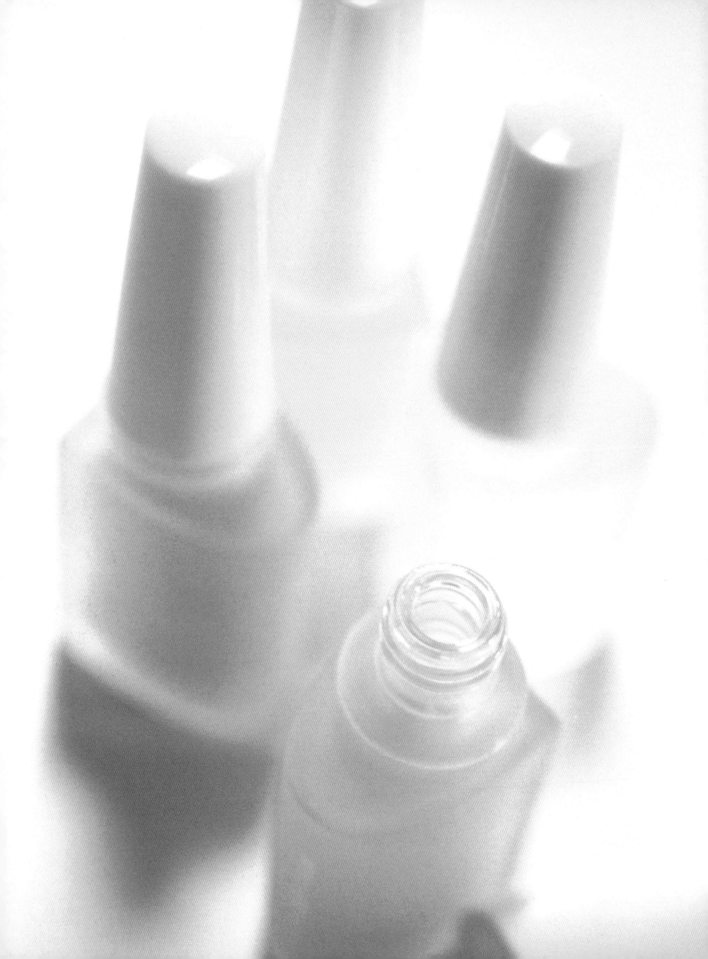

5

Nails

PRO POINTERS

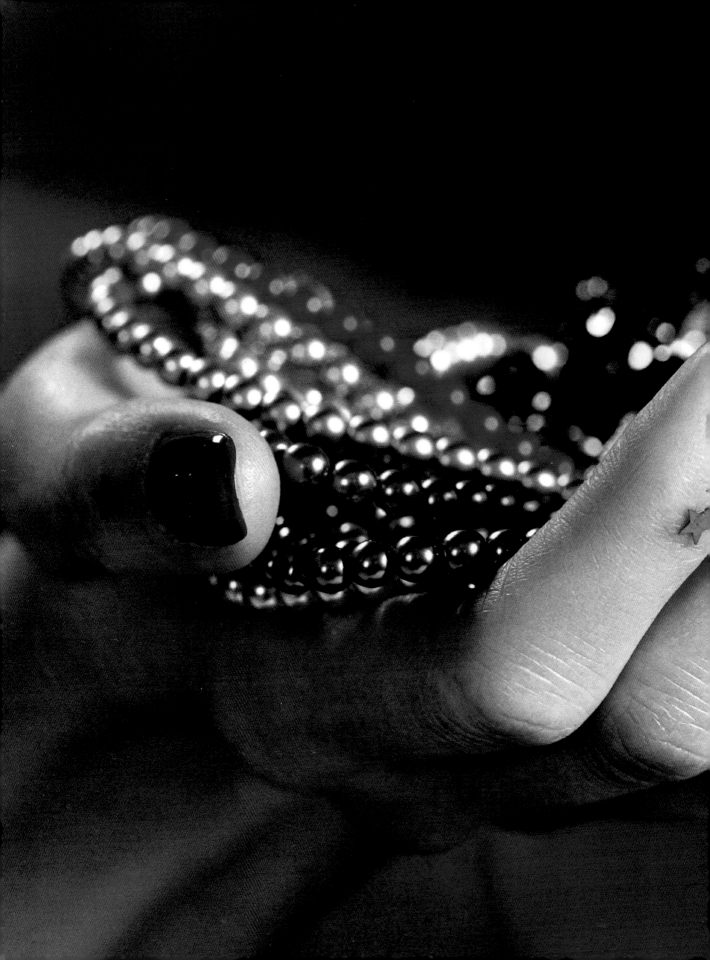

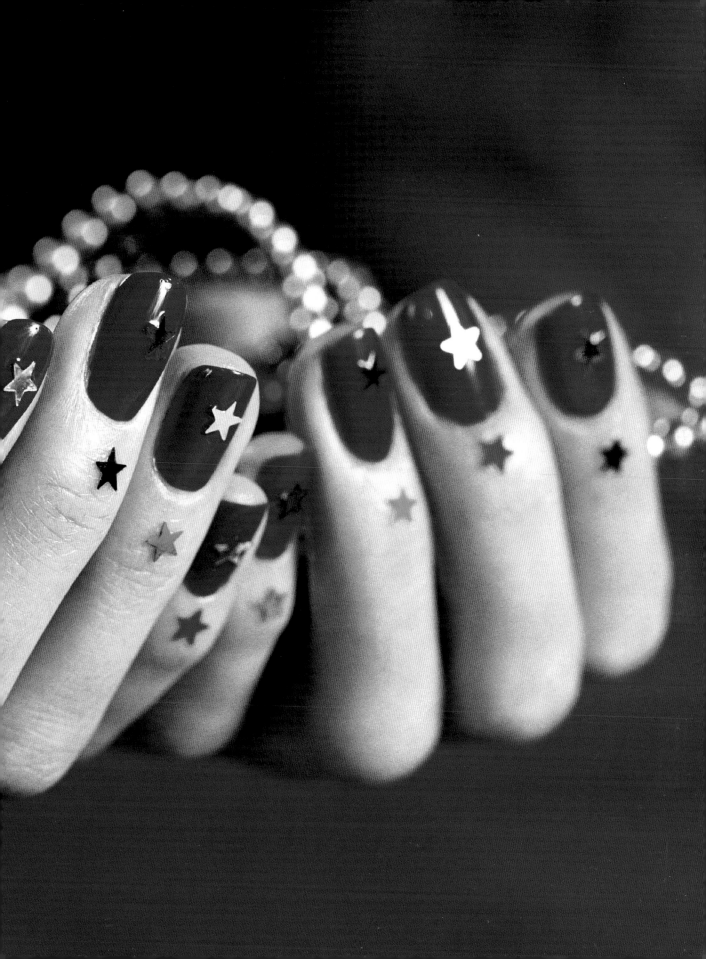

Poppies, pinks, and pastels: a perfect pretty palette

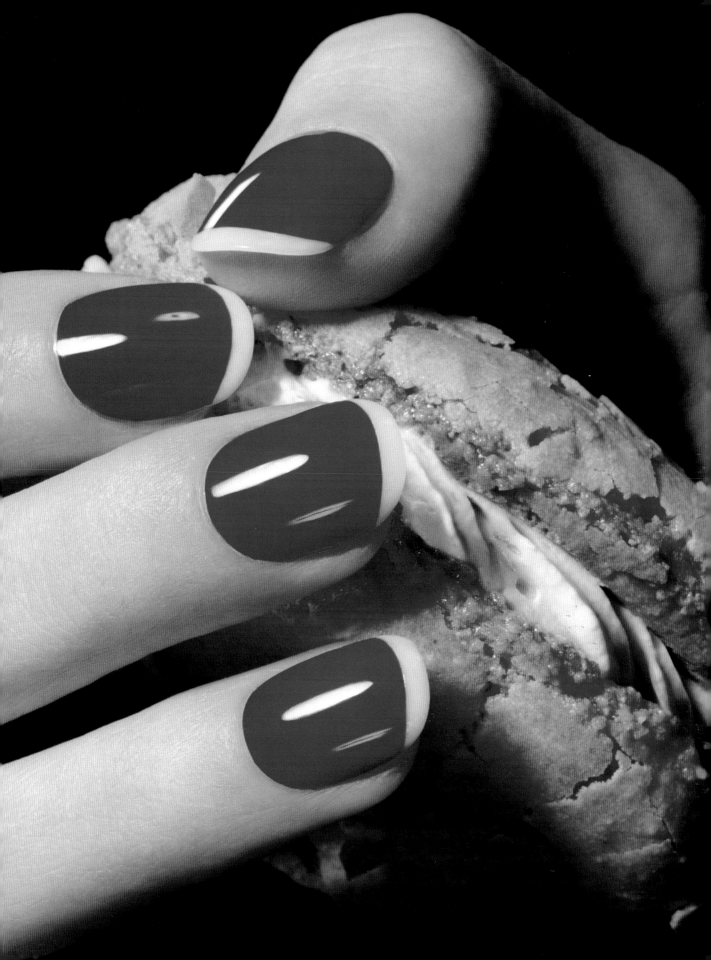

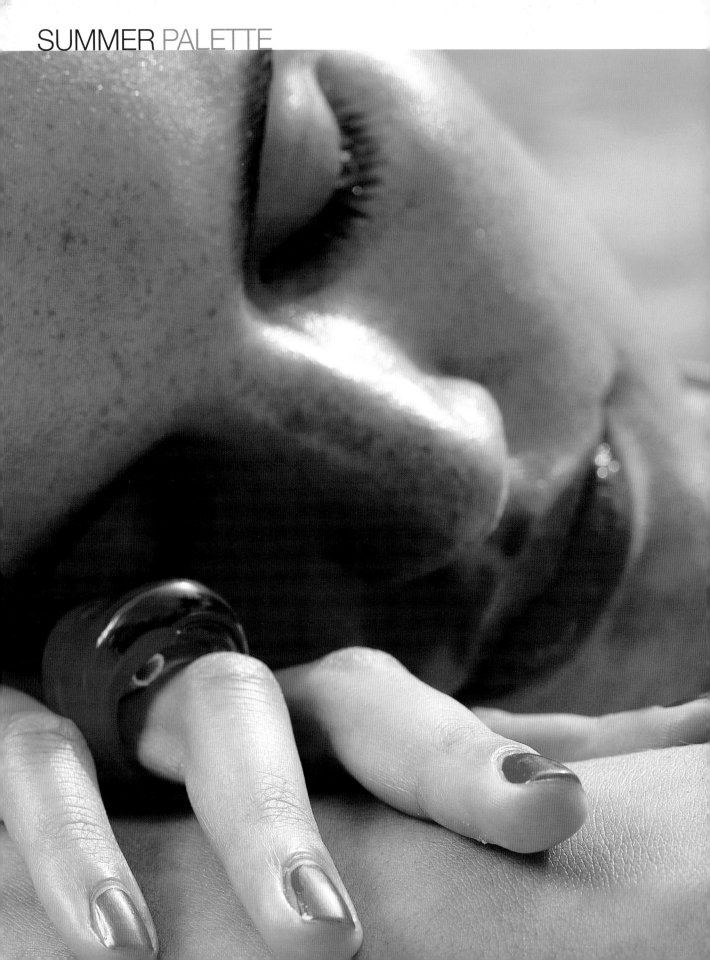

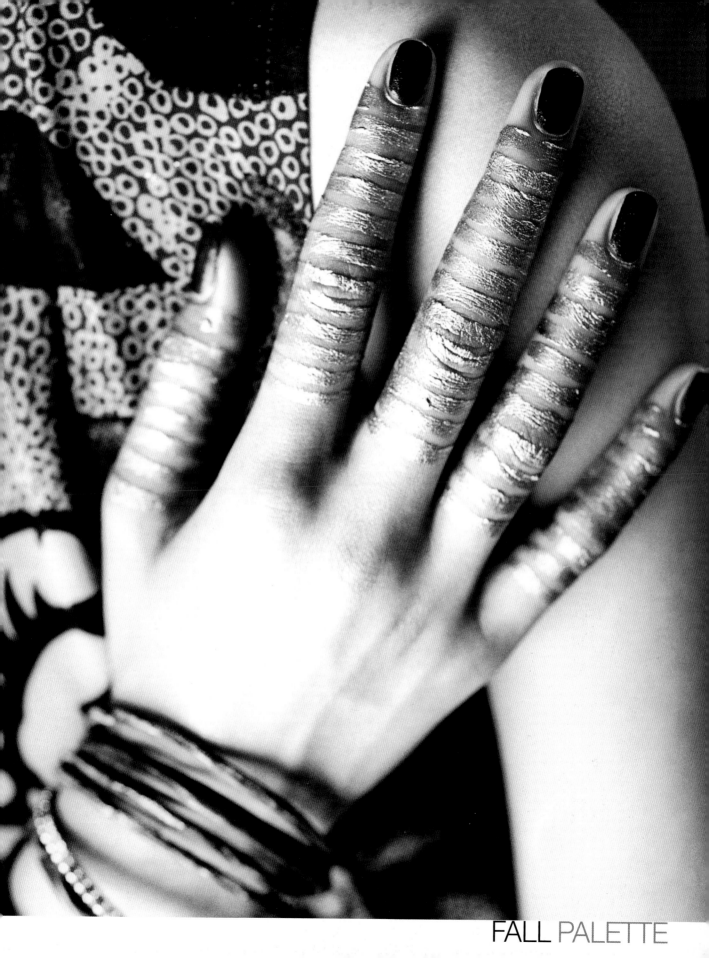

FALL PALETTE

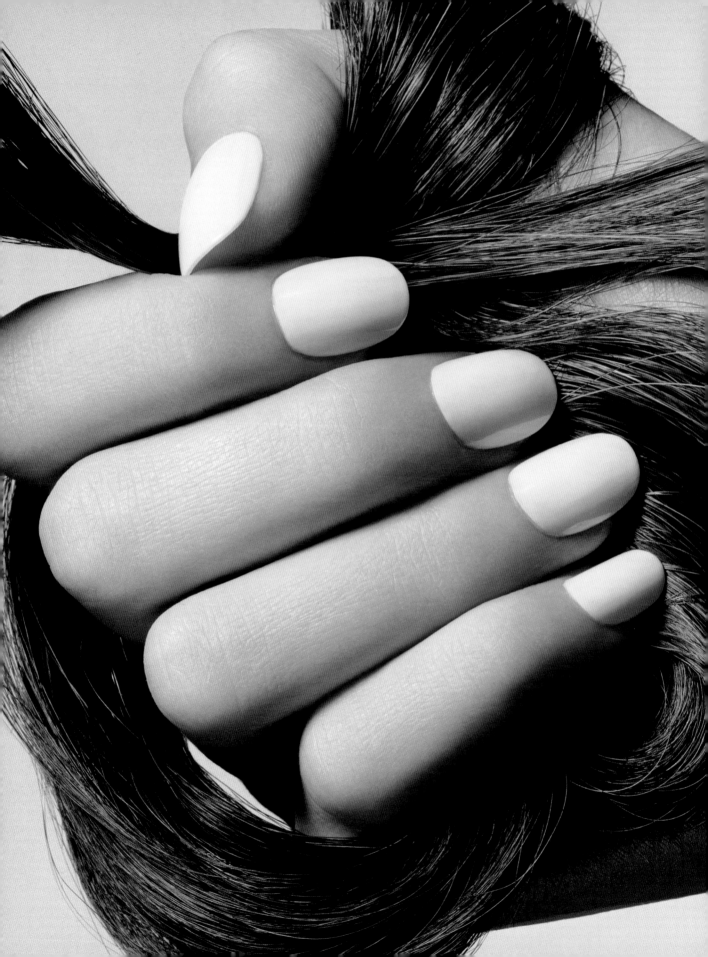

Pretty city girls prowling around town with style and flair

Express manicure

Nails are anything but simple accessories: chic or shocking, they arm your hands with an undeniable power of seduction.

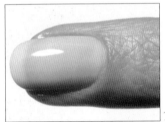

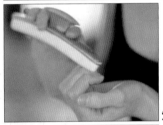

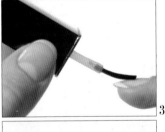

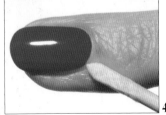

1 The key to beautiful nails lies in **CONSTANT CARE.** Cuticles should be pushed back and the smallest imperfection taken care of immediately. Daily use of the right nourishing and hydrating cream according to your skin type and age will help. The perfect length? Not too long and not too short. Use the shape of your fingertip as a guide to create a classic rounded square shape.

2 Your nails should be **FILED AS WELL AS BUFFED**. Whether or not you're going to use polish, the slightest bump will stick out like a sore thumb!

3 A **GOOD BASE AND PRIMER** will strengthen and protect your nails.

4 With today's products offering ultra-shiny and incredibly vibrant colors at record-breaking drying speed, beautiful nails have never been easier. **LET YOURSELF LOOSE!** However, beware of flaking and peeling: nothing looks more neglected than chipped nail polish.

ADVICE FROM A PROFESSIONAL NAIL CARE SPECIALIST GISÈLE POMMIER (L'onglerie)
With one sweep, take just enough polish for one nail and wipe any excess away into the bottle. Contrary to what most people believe, you should start in the middle of your nail, at the edge, fanning downward to the base, finishing at the sides, leaving a small space on either side.

What you'll need

- orangewood cuticle sticks
- nail file (emery board, glass, or ceramic)
- pumice stone
- manicure scissors
- nail clippers
- buffer
- exfoliating cream
- nourishing cream
- nail polish remover
- base and primer, nail polish, top coat, and activating spray

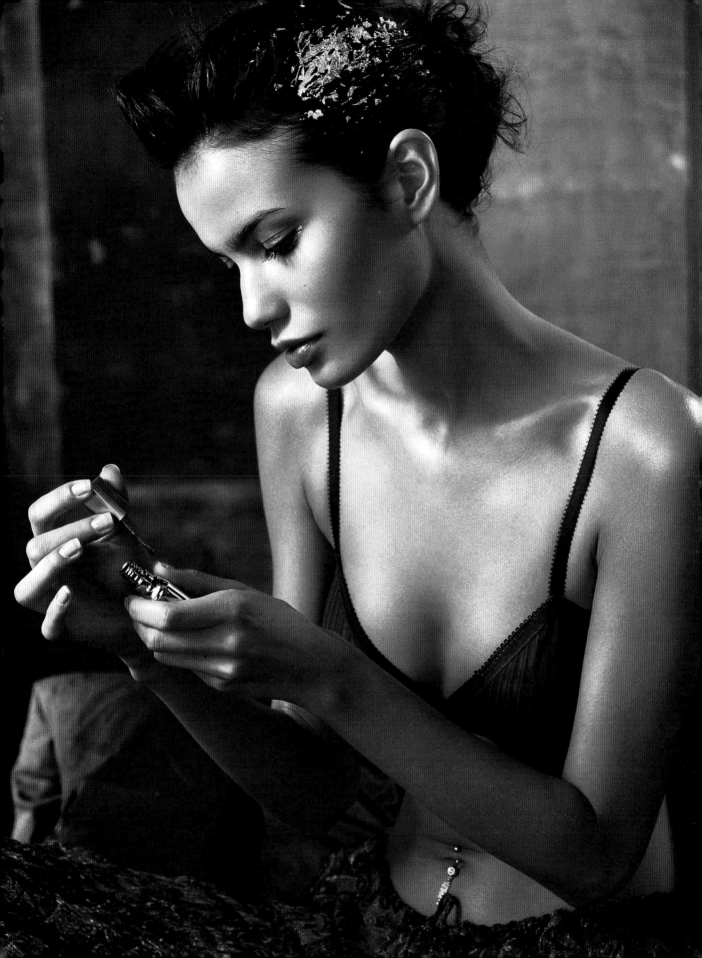

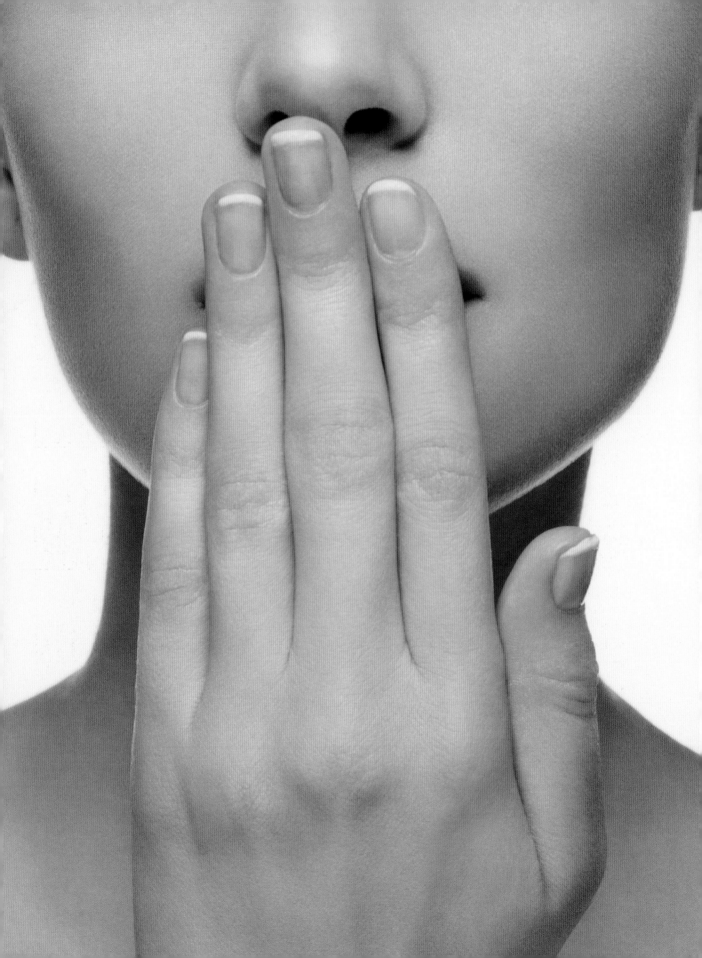

French manicure: A worldwide winner

Refined and flattering, this most famous of manicures requires care and attention to detail. Here are some tips to get you on the right track.

1 FILE THE NAIL rather short, once completely cleaned of old polish, either in a slightly squared or round shape.

2 REMOVE HANGNAILS with cuticle scissors—dead skin only. After applying a cuticle softening cream, push your cuticles back with a wood cuticle stick.

3 Delicately **APPLY WHITE POLISH** to nail tips, following the natural tip of the nails. You can try adhesive guide strips or a kit with a curved brush: any excess polish can be removed with a nail polish remover stick.

4 APPLY BEIGE OR PINK POLISH as soon as the opaque polish on the tips has completely dried. Cover your entire nail with clear polish, which will give the white tips a more natural look. Once you've got the hang of it, you can try to give yourself a colored French manicure or replace the white tips with gold or silver for a party.

5 A TOP COAT that protects while it shines is the last touch for an impeccable finish. It will also help increase the durability of your manicure. Top it off with a nourishing cream or oil.

ADVICE FROM ODILE SIBUET (manicurist)
French manicure kits are extremely practical: covering the nail plate, they leave just the tips exposed, helping you paint a perfect half-moon. Wait until the white polish is completely dry before removing the tip guide.

What you'll need
- nail file
- orangewood cuticle sticks
- cuticle cream
- white opaque polish
- beige or pink nail polish

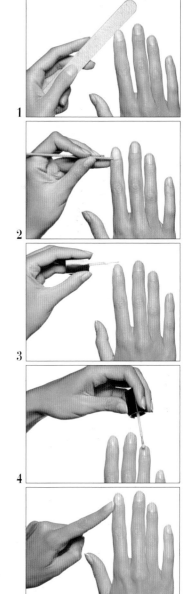

1

2

3

4

5

Your best foot forward

As soon as the sun comes out, you break out your sandals and show off your toes. Here are a few tips for beautiful feet from an expert podiatrist and pedicurist.

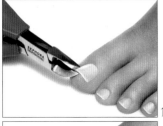

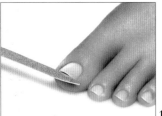

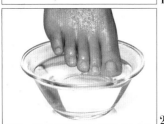

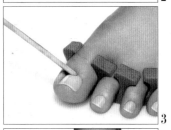

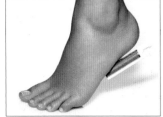

1 **TRIM** your toenails with clippers and even them into a rounded square shape with a nail file. Beware of cutting the corners too short, as this can lead to ingrown nails.

2 **EXFOLIATE THEN SOAK** your feet for 10 minutes in a warm bath of aromatherapy oils, bath balls, or Epsom salts. Use this time to scrub your toenails.

3 As soon as you remove your foot from the bath, **PUSH BACK** your cuticles with an orangewood cuticle stick. Next, buff your nails with a fairly abrasive buffer and then apply nail oil to the whole nail, paying particular attention to the nail bed.

4 Use a foot file or a wet pumice stone to **SLOUGH AWAY** calluses and dead skin cells on the balls and heels of your feet. To address corns and more serious foot issues, make an appointment with your podiatrist!

5 Give yourself a long **MASSAGE** using your favorite moisturizer. Using a cotton swab dipped in nail polish remover, get rid of any greasy residue on your toes. You're now ready to attempt a French pedicure!

ADVICE FROM ARI DARMON (Podiatrist and pedicurist)
Using an at-home foot spa with rollers will add to the relaxing aspect of your pedicure. Even without polish, your toenails can shine with a "supershine" buffer. Wrapping a bit of cotton on the end of your cuticle sticks will make pushing skin back less painful and, if dipped in nail polish remover, will also help you clean up after any application errors. To separate your toes, use a rolled-up facial tissue: it's practical and hygienic. Be sure to always dry between your toes to avoid cracks and fungal infections. Finally, put on your pedicure slippers before you start painting your toenails!

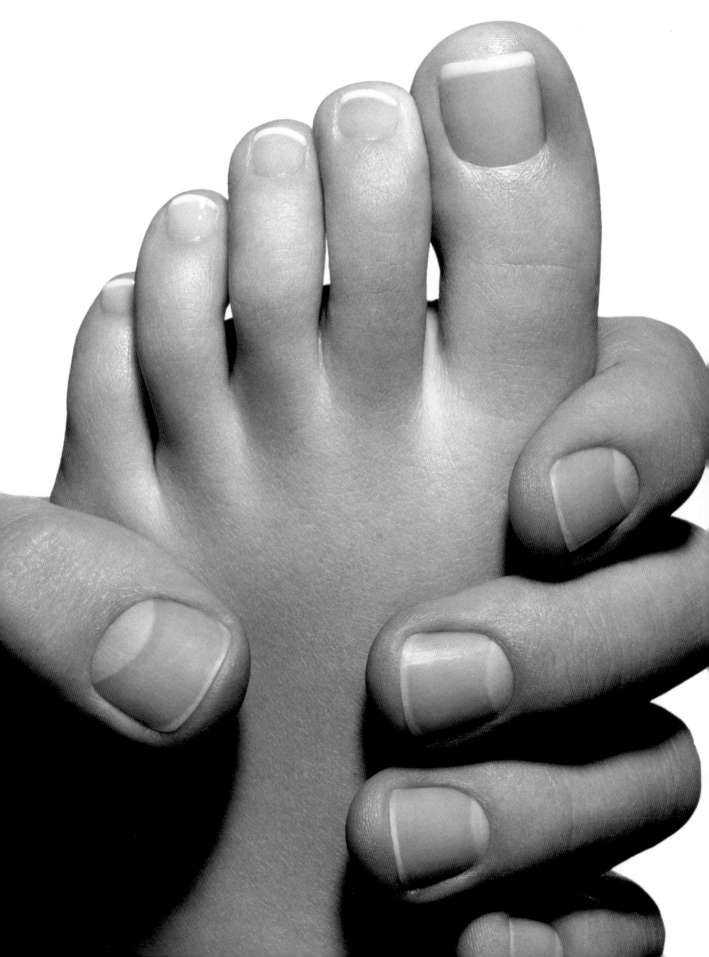

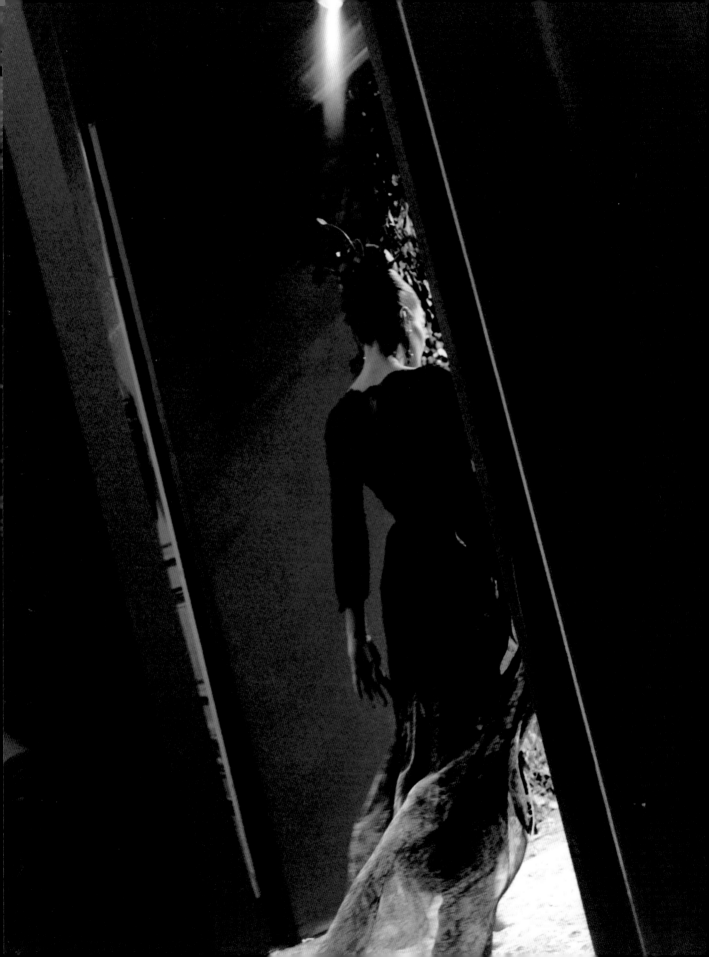

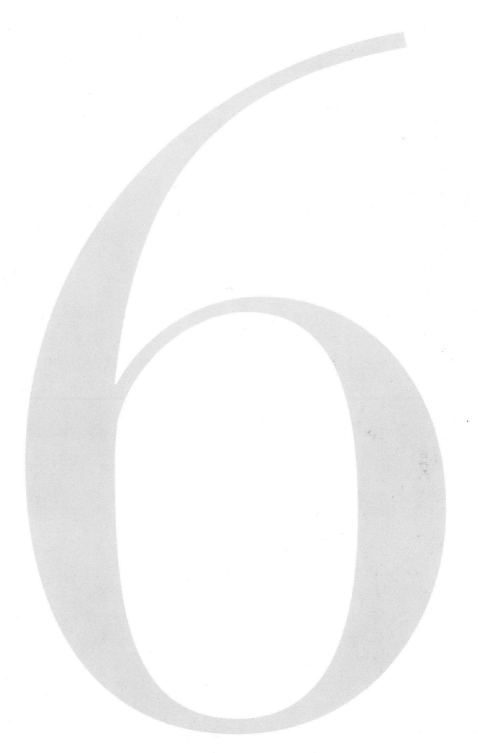

MAKEUP ARTISTS' SECRETS

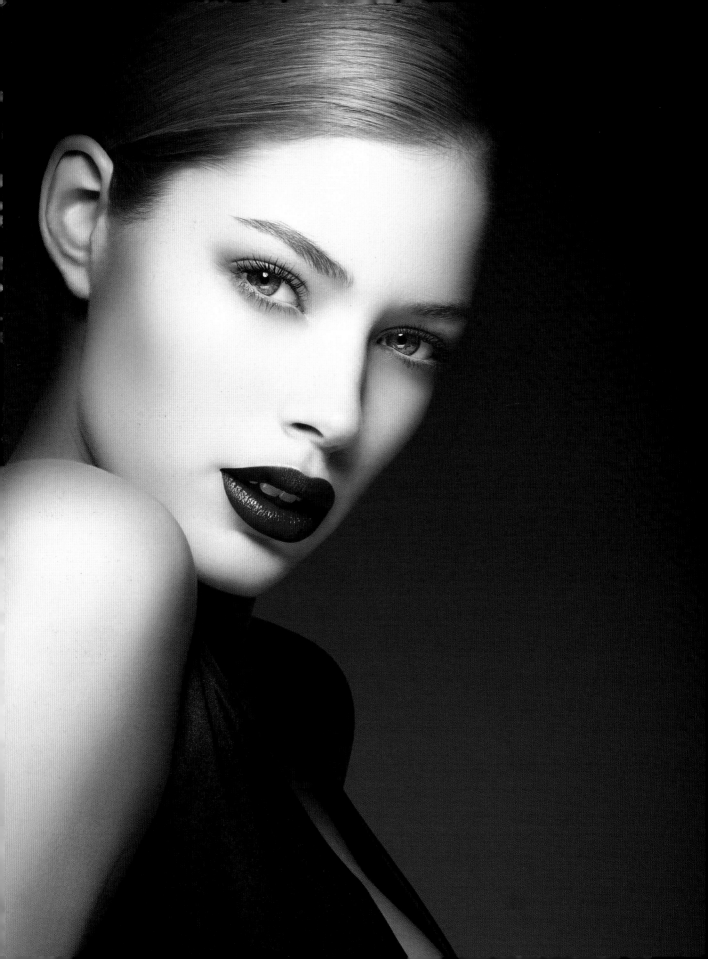

Olivier Échaudemaison

Creative Director, Guerlain

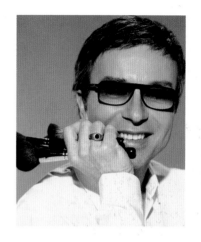

A makeup artist whose address book would make any celebrity watcher go green with envy, Olivier Échaudemaison is adored by queens, princesses, and celebrities the world over. His take on beauty is a lesson in the rules of attraction.

"The one thing to bring to a desert island? Lipstick!"

"Beauty is a timeless concept; it has nothing to do with short-lived trends or fads. That is why I prefer to talk about style rather than fashion. So why change when you've found yours? Trying to look like someone else is proof of insecurity, but today, we don't know how to look at ourselves anymore; we see ourselves only in pieces. It's time to rediscover an overall vision of ourselves. This is why I love "before and after" makeovers—the only problem is when the "before" is better than the "after"! But seeing the same woman worked on by four different makeup artists, for example, would be a dream…

In my 40 years in the makeup industry, in spite of all the new gadgets, nothing has really changed: we still have eyes and lips. **How you wear your eyeliner or your lipstick is reassuring and self-affirming. After all, you're naked without it!**

Cosmetic products are only as interesting as the stories they tell: How do they seduce and attract all the senses? How aesthetically pleasing are they? How sensuous to the touch? Even the sounds of the clasps and the smell of perfumes count.

Without spending too much, you can indulge in boundless luxury, self-gratification, and a certain social status associated with projecting a strong image.

On the other hand, what has changed are the formulas and the ways we apply makeup: the invention of weightlessness and radiance. Guerlain has illustrated this trend with the creation of Meteorites and especially Terracotta, a 20-year-old revolution: makeup that you can't see.

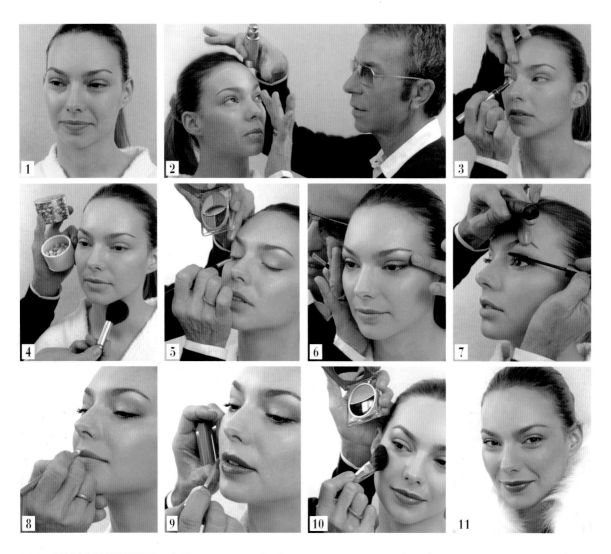

MID-SEASON MAKEUP. **1.** Use an intense hydrating cream on your clean face. **2.** Use moisturizing foundation for a natural and flawless complexion. **3.** Apply stick concealer in the inner corner under your eye. For more effective blending with your skin, smooth concealer with your fingertips from the inner to the outer corner. **4.** For a superb complexion, use a facial powder with hints of gold and mother-of-pearl. These bring a harmonious radiance and translucency. Brighten your complexion by dipping the brush in the powder and applying over the whole face, neck, and shoulders, paying particular attention to the nose, chin, and forehead. **5.** Apply beige eyeshadow to create a mysterious look. **6.** Voila! Larger eyes. **7.** Final (and indispensable) step for your eyes: mascara. This will give depth and volume to your lashes. **8.** Use lip pencil to highlight the cupid's arrow of your upper lip. **9.** For a shiny, lacquered effect, use lipstick or gloss with a shiny finish. **10.** Blush is the final touch, after applying your lipstick. **11. The result: makeup that is both soft and sophisticated.**

"By watching Ava Gardner onscreen, women could borrow a beauty recipe or two!"

When a woman says, "I don't use makeup; I just use Terracotta," it makes me laugh! This spectacular technological revolution is to makeup what microfibers and spandex were to fashion.

What this means for you is that you don't have to be an expert anymore to do your own makeup.

Years ago, cosmetics were hard to work with, and women made mistakes. It was a difficult art, reserved for a precious few, such as actresses and socialites. Besides these and other worldly women, who got made up professionally, few women could afford such luxury.

Nevertheless, since time immemorial, women have found solutions. They soon realized that as far as beauty is concerned, all you need is a good recipe and good examples! While admiring such great performers as Ava Gardner, women were able to borrow a trick or two for themselves. ▶

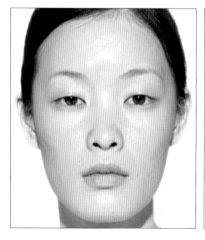 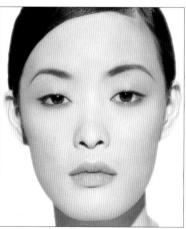 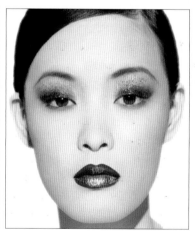

HEIN, STYLED BY OLIVIER ÉCHAUDEMAISON in three spectacular steps: **1.** Before. **2.** For daytime: a foundation that creates a seamless complexion, eyebrows redrawn with a pencil, eyes highlighted with beige eyeshadow and lifted by a touch of black eyeliner, shiny rose lipstick. **3.** For evening: glitter and more daring colors for shadow; a touch of lip liner, lipstick, and a dash of blush give the final accents. ▶

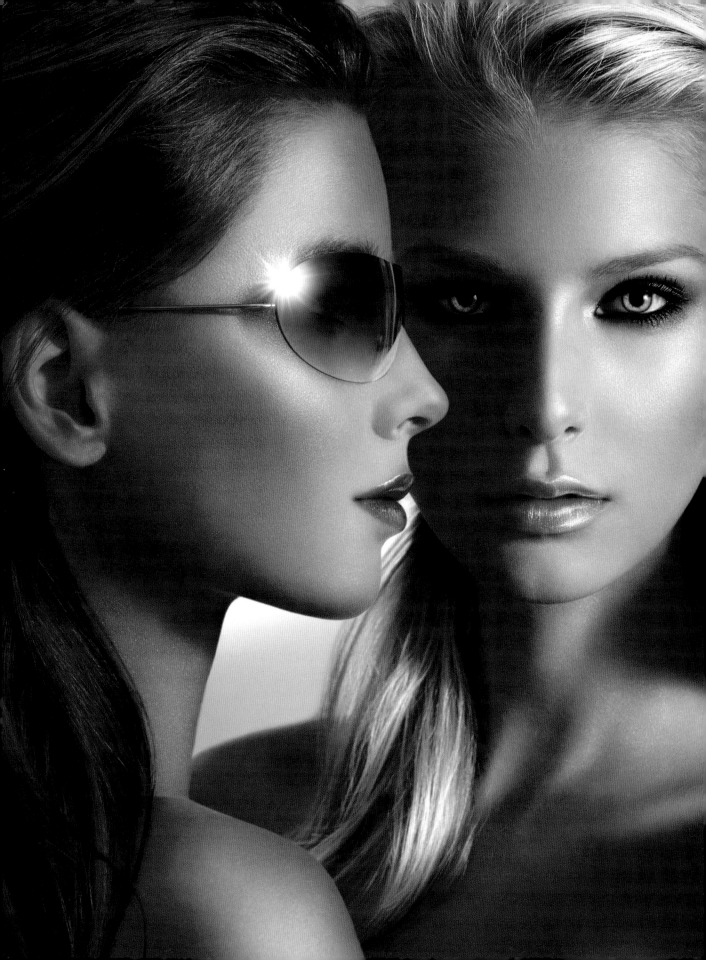

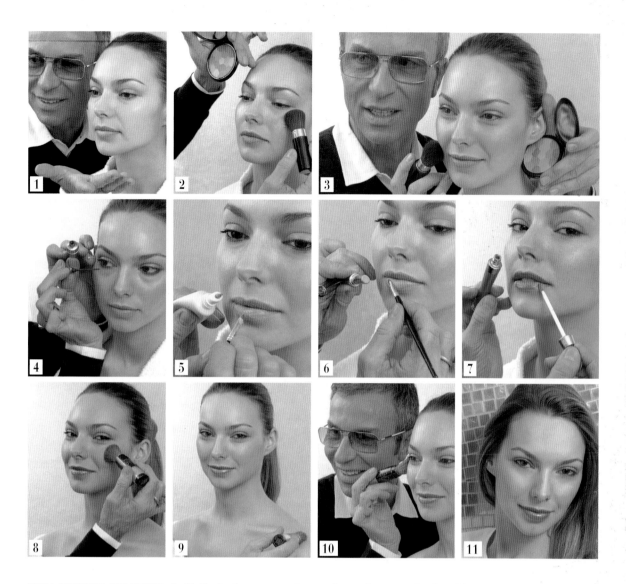

SUN-KISSED BEAUTY. 1. Fully hydrate your skin with a gel-cream. **2.** To add a sun-kissed radiance to your face and highlight certain features, such as your cheekbones or your eyebrow arch, apply bronzing powder with a brush. **3.** Simply beautiful: a bright and natural complexion. **4.** For a captivating, sensual, and downright fascinating look, use kohl liner which can be applied on the eyelid as well as on the inner lower lid. Easy to wear, it opens up the expressions of blondes and brunettes alike without hardening your face; it simply leaves you mysteriously sexy. **5.** For perfectly moisturized lips, use a brush to apply lip balm before lipstick or gloss. **6.** To prep your lips for lipstick and ensure long-lasting color, use a lipstick base or some concealer. **7.** For a soft and radiant smile, choose a glossy hue. **8.** An amber shade blush makes your tan effervescent. **9.** For a sensual glow, caress your face and body with highlighting powder. **10.** To get people to pay attention to you, apply to strategic zones, such as your neck, shoulders, arms, and ankles. **11.** A bright sun-kissed look that lasts for hours. **Result, on the opposite page: a sun-kissed face and body,** composed of brown, copper, and golden nuances.

▶

"Foundation is as intimate as lingerie— as close to your skin as it gets."

Neutral is the name of the game: from foundation to lipstick. Today's makeup is elusive—secret and imperceptible. If you can see the work that goes into it, then you haven't succeeded…

Foundation is as intimate as lingerie—as close to your skin as it gets. If it's poorly chosen, it can look terrible. What's more (and this is what makes product development so fascinating these days), it can just as well be practically invisible today. **People shouldn't say to you, "What a lovely foundation you're wearing today!" but rather, "Your skin looks beautiful today!"**

As for your lips, they can live their own life—red, purple, or gothic black—because they show the color of your mood. They also affirm your sensuality, not to mention your sexuality: men won't ever put makeup on their lips!

Lips have always been a fashion accessory: during the miniskirt craze of the 1960s, leggings were yogurt-colored and lips were pearly white to compensate up for the sexed-up leg exposure. It was a way of toning down any sexual connotation of the lips. In the 1970s, when mid-length and long skirts came back into style, lips were done in copper and brown!

A pants-wearing woman without makeup could be considered masculine. But the same woman, in the same outfit with heels and red lips is a knockout!

The one thing to bring to a desert island? Lipstick! And that's it!

A fetishistic object, lipstick is an incredible weapon of seduction. If a woman chooses to use it in public, and if the act of using it is beautiful to behold, the object itself must be as well. KissKiss, Guerlain's signature lipstick that I reintroduced to the market with Van Straten's help, is timeless and sensual. It's unbelievable to think that it has conquered 17% of the worldwide cosmetic market!

Women are attracted to its name, its color, and its shape. We're not talking about consumerism. We're talking about instinct and pure pleasure.

*A snow princess straig
out of a fairytale showcas
a winter palett*

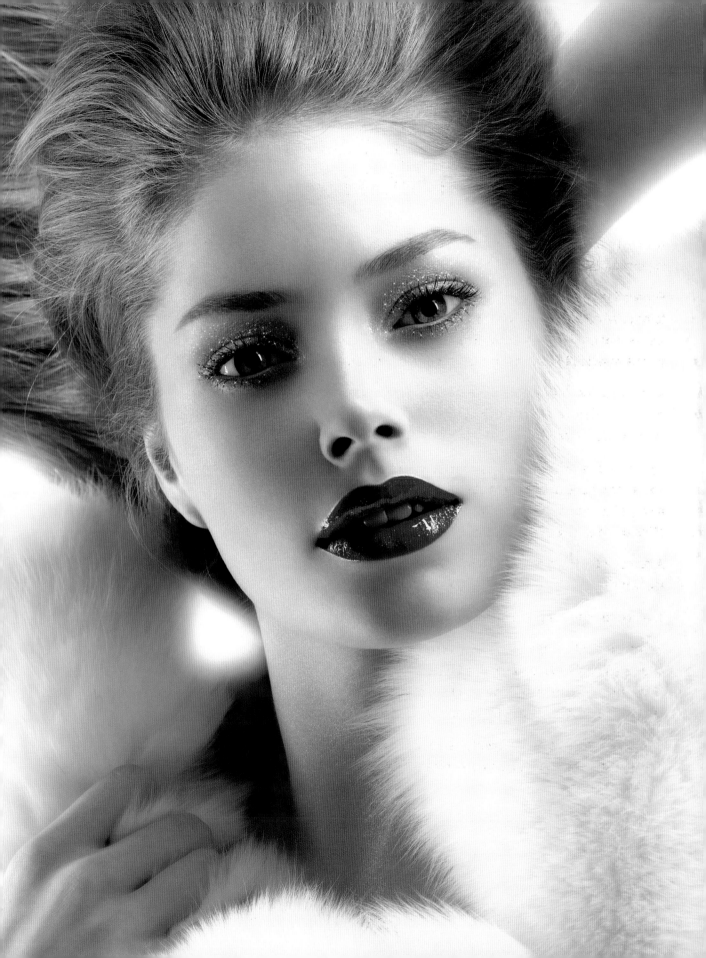

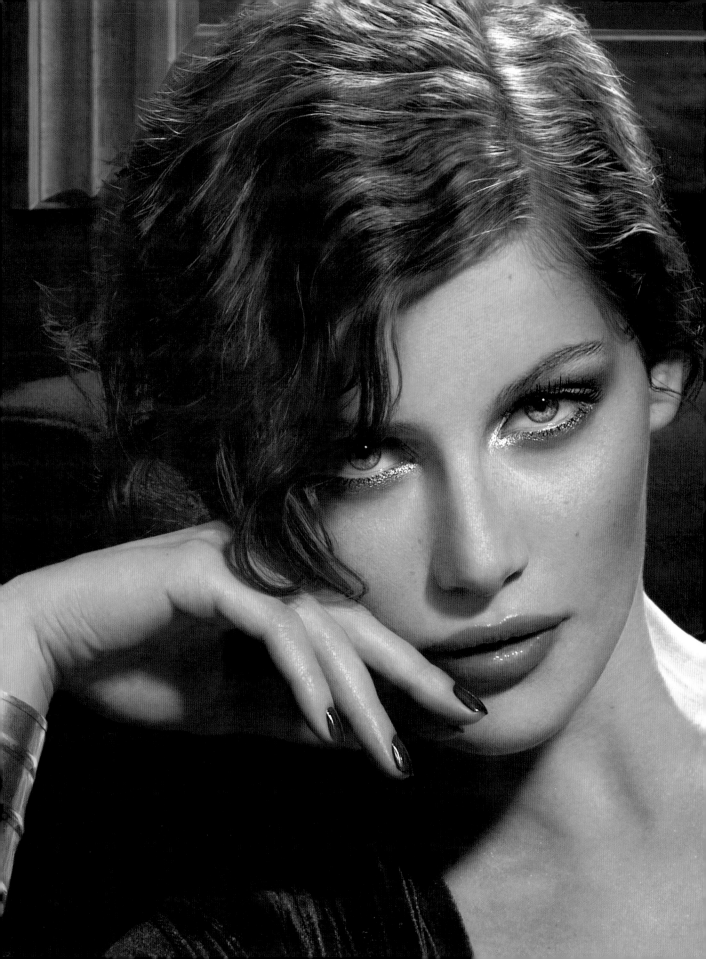

James Kaliardos
Makeup Artist at L'Oréal Paris

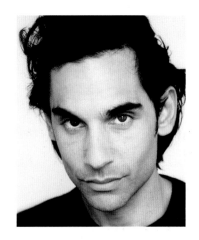

James Kaliardos is an artist of feeling: he holds the women he makes up in high esteem and is interested in each person as a whole. Whether she is unknown or world-renowned, he conquers every woman he works on thanks to his luminous art that exists somewhere between spectacular and natural. Each perfect detail contributes to one singular image that is always sublime.

"Makeup is a powerful way to effectively reveal something unique about your inner self"...

"Nothing forces a woman to make herself up or have her hair done—these are only means to an end—powerful ways to effectively reveal something unique about your inner self to give you the necessary confidence to express yourself.

Clearly there has been a revolution around how women relate to beauty—I am currently working on a project where I study the changes in the role of beauty in women's lives during each decade. I already had some ideas of what these changes meant, but I did not understand the fundamental reasons behind them. For example, throughout history, as wars have broken out, women have been pushed "behind the scenes." At war's end, they come back to the forefront, feeling the need to have a certain type of look that is often rather extreme.

We're lucky today to be living in a time of freedom where women can actually choose how they want to look. Makeup can be "trendy," not wearing it can be, too. Wearing your hair straight is in vogue as much a tousled, straight-out-of-bed look.

Women living in the 1950s were forced into conformity by wearing thick foundation, red lipstick, and eyeliner. They also often got perms at the hairdresser. In short, fashion was dictated, and unfortunately, the accepted standard did not work for everyone!

▶

Laetitia Casta, the ultimate muse,
is the epitome of ideal beauty.

"Your 'look' only counts for 20%. What's essential is your personality, your way of being…"

Now imagine yourself in the '60s: you would need an extra half-hour per day to put on your false eyelashes. Men have never had these types of constraints.

All that is over now—today, you can do as you please! This represents true power for today's women—a crucial victory, even though we must not forget that in some places of the world, women are not allowed to show their faces.

Sometimes I work on photo shoots where the models are treated horribly, posing in a dark alley or on a staircase like some poor streetwalker. I am ferociously against that. In fashion, we work with the world's most beautiful women; is it really necessary to show them in this light? I fight constantly against these types of images and believe in more noble representations of women. **A woman can be truly strong and beautiful at the same time. I think that beauty is a power that men will never have.** Women have their own particular sensitivity; they have a direct access to their feelings that are unique to them, and such strength of character can, I believe, help change the world.

Beauty, like fashion, is a question of choice. With just one model, you can create an infinite number of

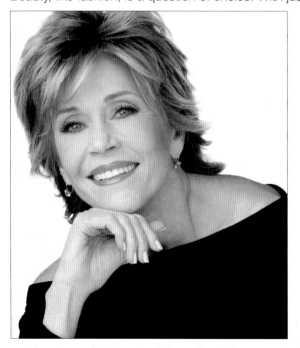

photos…working with her personality, you can invent the role that she will play in the final product. A shocking mane or straightened locks, infinitely long eyelashes or the reddest lips, high heels or sneakers: the possibilities are endless.

When I meet a woman for the first time, I, of course, notice her makeup, but I try to see first and foremost what kind of person she is. ▶

I love **Jane Fonda's** recent films. They are so full of emotion and depth! Being beautiful is not about throwing your hair around rapturously (laughing). The foundation you see here, Age Re-Perfect, was invented for mature skin—women over 60—and I love it so much that I use it on 16-year-old girls!

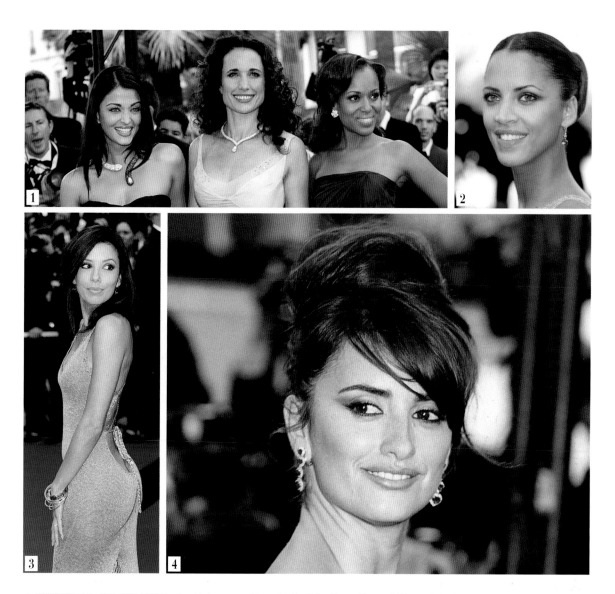

A FESTIVAL OF CHARM. 1. Aishwarya Rai, Andie MacDowell, and Kerry Washington **2.** Noémie Lenoir **3.** Eva Longoria **4.** Penélope Cruz. Many think—wrongly—that the beauty world is artificial, superficial: I never stop fighting against such stereotypes and always try to inject it with authenticity… Even if everything we do is based on technique, we really do try to bring another dimension to beauty. And doing this is all the more simple with L'Oréal Paris **since our ambassadors are not only unbelievably beautiful but they also have equally unbelievable personalities.** They were in fact all chosen primarily for their personality and not just for their stunning physical traits: their looks only count about 20% in our decision. The rest lies in their manner of expressing themselves, what they represent—and that's what makes them amazing women. My mission is to help out in the fascinating crossroads that is the Cannes Film Festival, where two worlds coexist. Attending the festival is a huge inspiration—there is so much respect for artistic creation. I find it immensely moving when people jump out of their seats to clap at the end of a film. This festival gives great credit to the artists' work: moviegoers look beyond the "entertainment" aspect of a film and acknowledge the immense amount of work that goes into its making. It's a miraculous thing, and what makes cinema delightful is that we see ourselves on-screen… **The beauty of actresses affects us like a dream**—there is that astonishing relationship between stars and fans, those countless declarations of love as they walk the length of the red carpet…

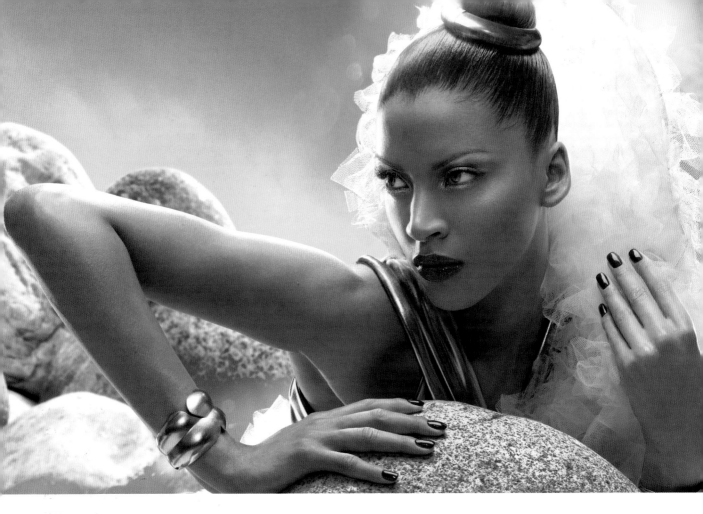

The same goes for photo shoots—I drown in the image that the model is transmitting and in the personality that she is offering to the world. Moreover, my work consists in never-ending choices to be made (okay, enough porcelain skin, let's move on!) The way you do your own hair or makeup is a choice and should be seen as a way of making a statement about yourself. Beware, though, of falling into a routine. **It's important to rethink your look from time to time, to "break with tradition" and try something new** that really works for you. You don't look the same at 20, 40, or 60… As you grow older, you adapt and evolve as your looks change. There is nothing sad about this "beauty evolution." *Au contraire!* Listen to the advice of your beauty professionals for a new hair style, for example. I do the same thing: when I don't know what to wear, I ask my stylist friends! Get your makeup done at a makeup counter: you don't have to buy a thing, and if you don't like the results, you can wash it off! Above all, look around you, keep your eyes open: there is so much to absorb! Get inspiration from magazines (or the pages of this book!), and you'll discover what you're naturally attracted to. It's up to you afterward to determine what suits you best, if it's realistic, or if it's pure fantasy. If something looks like "you," go for it! Make yourself happy. There's only one way to (re)discover yourself: in a mirror, without makeup, as if you were looking at someone else.

Noémie Leno transfigured, surreal…

154

"There is only one way to (re)discover yourself: in a mirror, without makeup, as if you were looking at someone else!"

Just one rule: avoid taking a sudden dislike to what you see. Focus rather on what you like, since that is what you're going to highlight… Take your eyes, for example: there are plenty of ways to play with eye makeup. So many products are available today, and you probably already spend much more on your hair than on your eyes. Take advantage of what's available. You never know, it might just change your life. Set up "beauty meetings" with your girlfriends—my mother did it; there were always women around the house getting their hair done.

What's the real secret? Light. It's fundamental to beauty. You can do the most beautiful makeup imaginable, but if you are in the wrong light, it can look awful. Mirrors aren't the most important makeup accessory, it's your lighting. That's what will show you how you'll look to others. If you say to yourself, "Oh no! That's not me," when you see yourself in a mirror during the day or in a picture, then something's gone wrong. Don't hesitate to leave the warm light of your bathroom to check your makeup in daylight or under a harsh fluorescent light. It's worth a walk to the window to find the right foundation or eyeshadow!

JAMES AND HIS STARS

Some women know exactly how they want to look. **Angelina Jolie** is that way: a thin, dry black line along her brows and lipstick since she doesn't like the natural color of her lips. She chose gray and I refused to use it: I prefer beige! Making up Angelina was a dream; she is so intelligent and knows what she's doing. She artfully masters her round face—eyes, lips, and cheeks—by redrawing lines and creating a new structure. On the other hand, **Madonna** is more "Do what you like!" We tried tons of new stuff together. It was intoxicating, like a "work in progress." Both approaches are enjoyable for me, but I love working within strict limits. **Marilyn Manson** also knew precisely what look he wanted, and it was grandiose! My ego is never at play, I just go with the flow of each new situation. The most wonderful compliment I ever received was from **Richard Avedon:** "This kid's good!" I have had the immense privilege of working with some of the best photographers ever, like **Irving Penn** and **Helmut Newton.** They ushered me into their world and welcomed me: it was a fabulous gift. ▶

JAMES'S FIVE-MINUTE MAKEOVER

FOUNDATION Always start off with a day cream and don't be shy with it. Taking good care in cleansing and moisturizing your skin is the basis of good makeup. Next comes foundation. You'll choose one according to your skin type. I prefer foundations that cover well but that you can "work with" according to your needs. That said, new formulas are downright magical and look "real." Today's laboratories are doing incredible things. **What matters almost as much as the formula is how you apply your foundation.** Your hands must be sensitive, and you must learn to dab evenly. A common error is to apply foundation like a skin cream. Don't forget, foundation is something else entirely. Apply it in small pats on the very specific zones that need to be hidden most before delicately blending outward on your face. A good rule of thumb is to put a small amount on your hand and to dab lightly in order to achieve a seamlessly natural look and to **avoid those oh-so-disgraceful demarcation lines between your jaw and neck.** Start under your eyes and then move on to all the zones you want to cover: around your nose, on your chin—all the middle areas of your face. Next move from your cheekbones to your jaw, usually a naturally flawless zone, and blend toward your neck. I often see women doing the exact opposite, applying heavy foundation first on their cheeks and missing all the important areas altogether!

EYES Don't shy away from **eyelash curlers—they are fabulous tools** that I consider vital, especially if you use curling mascara! A dot of foundation on your eyelids will help prep them before applying makeup, regardless of the look you choose. If you want a clearly defined eyeliner, start with eyeshadow first, and then apply eyeliner to avoid any shadow or powder infractions. It also holds the shadow in place. On the other hand, if you're shooting for a more smudged effect, start with eyeliner and blend it into the eyeshadow that's going to cover it. **Accentuate your eyes by giving them structure...**and finish off with mascara. **CHEEKS** Use blush sparingly since your eyes are done up.
LIPS What you'll do depends on the overall look: maybe you just want some gloss. Your lips will help overall balance and provide a touch of shiny color to hallmark your final look—lipstick always makes women look more made up. **POWDER** The perfect happy ending: that final sweep across your T-zone provides dazzling confirmation that your makeup took only five minutes to apply—from cream to powder including eyes, lips, and cheeks! ▶

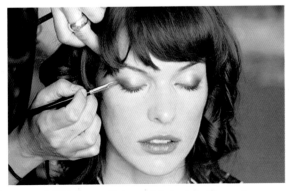
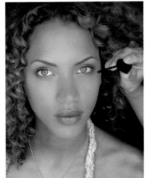
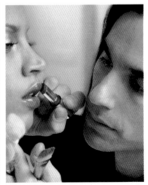

From Milla's eyelids to Noémie's lips, the same loving attention to detail.

Laetitia under James's masterful brush stroke.

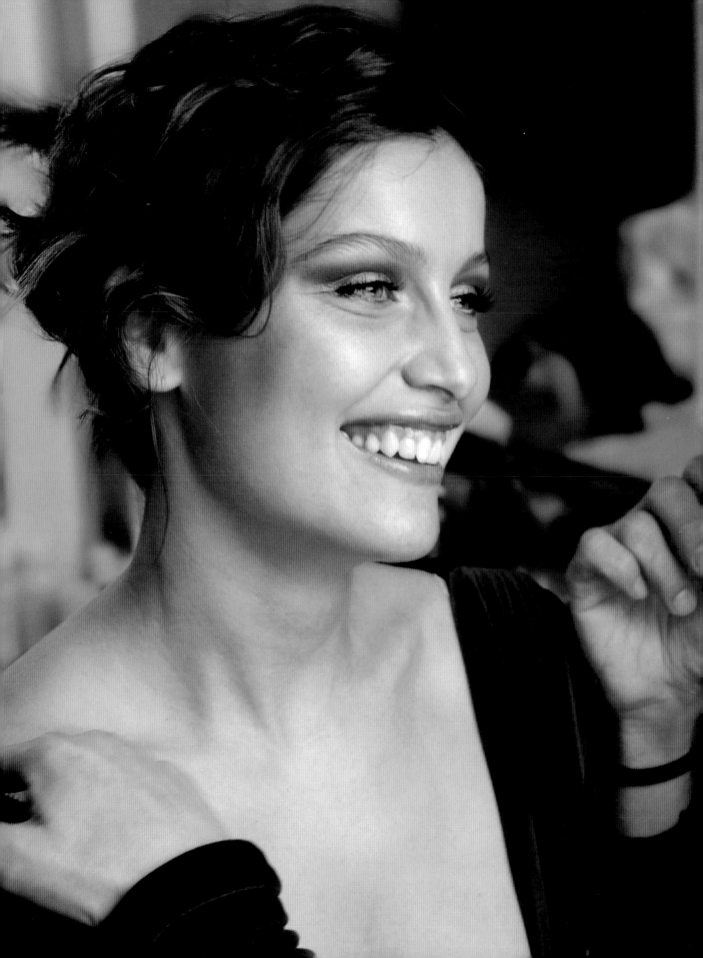

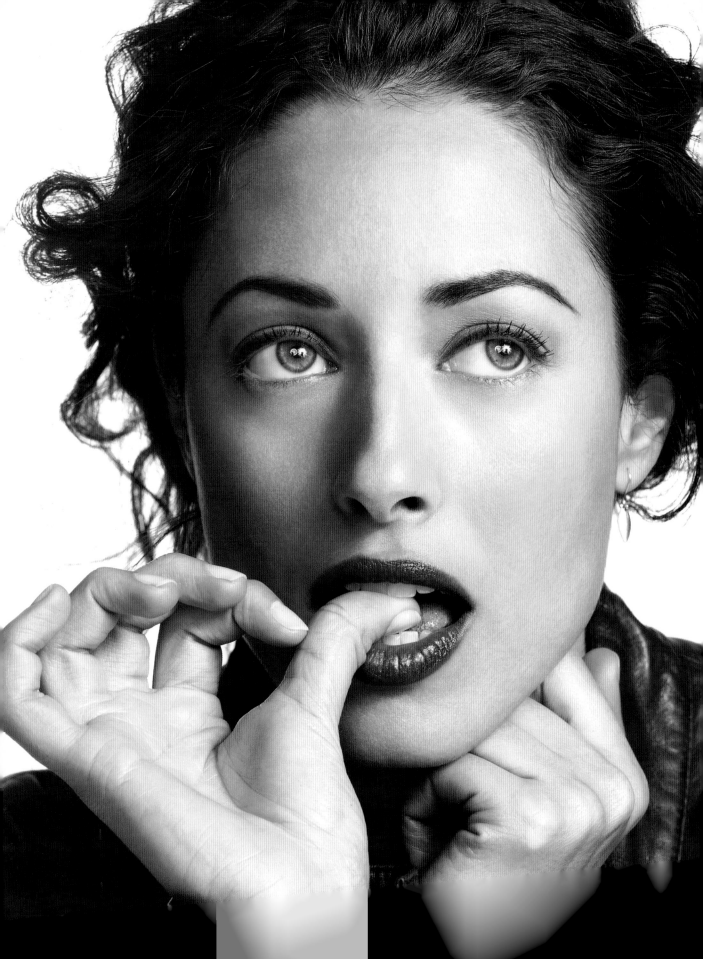

Bobbi Brown

Founder and C.E.O. of
Bobbi Brown Cosmetics

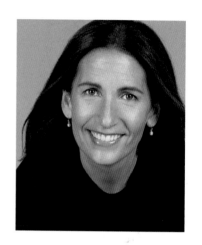

Bobbi Brown is one of a kind. With her unique, feel good approach to beauty, she holds her own in the highly selective club of celebrity makeup artists. Her motto? Be who you are. Her mission? Help every woman reclaim her own beauty.

"All I want is for my makeup to help make women happy!"

" I don't think that I'm particularly different—I simply think that I'm more in tune with ordinary women because I see myself in everyone. The top magazine models in glamorously sublime pictures simply don't reflect real life. Real life is where you just want to look pretty and bring out the best in yourself, starting every morning with what you've got. That type of "real life" is second-nature to me—and I'd love for that to be the case for all women! That's what I want to get across to women everywhere. "Beautiful" doesn't mean looking younger than you are; it just means looking great.

It's easy to think that beauty starts with your eyes or your mouth, but it really starts with your skin. Whether you have wrinkles or are barely 20, if you can achieve a seamless complexion without looking "made up," then you have what it takes. After all, it's their dreamlike skin that makes the top models so stunning…

I find it strange that you never see women over the age of thirty in the magazines. You can be inspired by the models even if you don't necessarily identify with them. **You want to know my approach to being yourself? Don't ever compare yourself to anyone. It's fine to admire but not to compete. You'll only wind up losing!** ▶

*Chocolate lip color—
a signature Bobbi look.*

"There's always a way to be your best you."

As a woman, I've always known what women wanted to look like, even top models. It is important to me that my products make women happy. That's rare in this business—most makeup artists don't care. For me, what matters is that women feel attractive, whether they are models or not. If I were working a show and the girls asked to take off their makeup as soon as they stepped off the podium, I'd take it as an insult.

At 20 you're sublime, but you don't know it. When I was that age, thrown into the high-fashion world fresh from my native Midwest, I didn't have the slightest idea.

It's hard to believe that you've "made it"—I've only felt that way for the past four years or so. **The secret? I don't try anymore to be something. I just am.** It's an unbelievably comfortable feeling, and people are always telling me how good I look, how refreshed, even at parties where I'm hanging around in jeans hobnobbing with top models (cheating a little with heels since I'm so short!)

If you try to be something you're not, it will never work.

Being yourself means taking hold of everything you can that will make you feel (and look) your best. And when being true to yourself, whatever the situation, there is always a way to be at your best—thanks to makeup!

Of course makeup is only part of a bigger package: taking care of yourself means eating well, drinking plenty of water—without forgetting that organic vegetables or other health foods can go well with a good glass of wine (for example, I think Chianti works perfectly with olive oil, dark chocolate, and green tea)—and not smoking. Let's not forget about choosing the right clothes, including the right underwear (it's impossible to feel great if they're not practical!)

And don't forget, makeup is not a question of what's trendy, but of personal style. You can find one that's right for you at any age. We've understood that in the cosmetics industry: when we've developed products that are right for you, we don't change them. That's the reasoning behind the permanence of our trademark lines.

I'm a makeup artist, and I love working on fashion shoots, brushing shoulders with the stars, and experimenting on them in the heat of the moment. All the same, when I see a woman for the first time, I see the person, not the makeup she's wearing. What I do notice, on the other hand, is when makeup is too harsh or too played up. Within moments of seeing a face for the first time, I know what it needs. My job, after all, is training makeup professionals! ▶

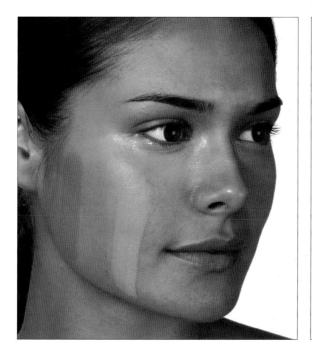
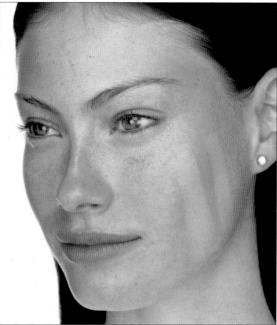

A TRICK TO FINDING THE PERFECT FOUNDATION. Try a stick, it's easier for testing (before settling on a different formula): apply three different shades on your lower cheek, and pat the three of them to find the right shade for you. Choose the one that you can barely see, that's neither oily nor yellow (and pick concealer one shade lighter).

BOBBI'S TOUCH IN 10 EASY STEPS

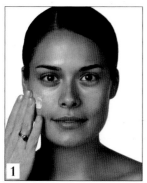
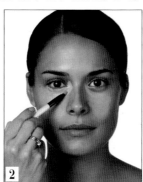
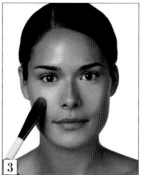
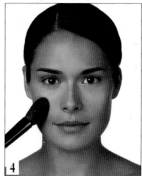

COMPLEXION. 1. If your skin is not correctly prepped, nothing will stick! Smooth moisturizer around your eyes before applying your concealer (so that it holds better). **2.** Applying corrector with a brush both neutralizes the shadows under your eyes and perks up your face. For bluish shadows under your eyes, use a rosy color. To protect the creamy base, dab gently up to the lash line and around your whole eye. **3.** Use a brush to apply a generous amount of under-eye concealer (too much comes out if you use your fingers). Trace a line around your eyebrows and gently wipe off any excess with your finger. ▶

BOBBI'S TOUCH IN 10 EASY STEPS

FOUNDATION. 4. (See previous page) Brushes allow for a lighter finish, but you have more control using your fingers. Use yellow undertones, never rose-toned ones. For normal to oily skin that tends to shine, massage and powder, then remove excess with a large brush. Lightly dot concealer with a blending brush. You can also use matte tanning powder (test on your shoulders or forearm) for a "sun-kissed" look. Blush, too, is a possibility: while smiling, accentuate your cheekbones using a down-and-outward movement to hit the areas where you naturally blush.

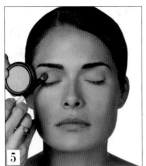 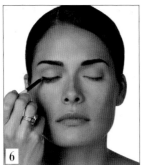 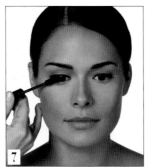 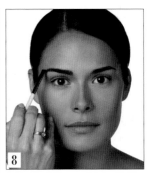

EYES. 5. For basic makeup: brush a matte color on your eyelid (tap away any excess). For a more sophisticated look: apply shadow onto the brush and then press on your hand so that the product penetrates deeply—correct with a blending brush and a cotton swab. Accentuate the eyes with a darker shadow, either dry or mixed with water, around the eye contours. **6.** Trace the baseline of your eye with an eyeliner pencil. Highlight only by filling in above the lash line, and don't try to modify its shape. Lightly pull your eyelid and fill in the roots of eyelashes (keep your swabs close!) Gel eyeliner, an exclusive of mine, does not run, is water-resistant, and easy to use. What's more, it glides on practically by itself. It provides a guaranteed optical illusion, like a second set of lashes, sober and elegant at the same time. **7.** Mascara: start from the roots and turn the brush as you pull it, like you would while drying your hair. Use a zigzag movement to create volume and thickening. **8.** Don't forget your eyebrows: use eyebrow mascara that's the natural color of your hair (or clear) for thicker brows and a bevelled-edge brush for thinner ones.

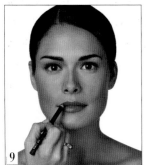 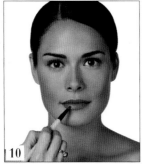 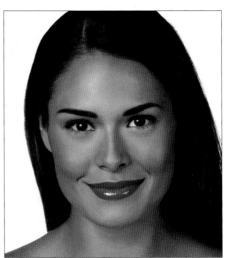

LIPS. 9. After lipstick application, use your lip liner for blending to maintain a natural appeal. **10.** Gloss will give your lips a smooth and softly radiant look. You can mix iridescent pinks with a matte tone. And why not a touch of lilac-infused gloss in the middle of your lips?

Manda as seen through Bobbi's eyes.

"Why have your eyelids redone? Just add some eyeliner."

How did I invent my eyeliner gel? I'm a very practical person. That day, I was in Colorado for a photo shoot (it was my picture being taken!) and, rifling through my bag, I realized I'd forgotten my eyeliner. I only had black mascara, and I used it to line my eyes and—surprise!—it held all day. I immediately called my office and said, "We're going to invent the first eyeliner that is ready for the long haul." That is how I work. Feeling good at any age means being in control—expending a little effort on your hair and makeup… I've never wanted to have my eyelids redone—all you need to do is add more eyeliner. Compulsive cosmetic surgery makes me sick: women never look younger or more beautiful; they just look like they've had something done. The more you're worried about your body, the more it shows on your face.

BOBBI AND HER STARS

As far as celebrities go, I adore **Jodie Foster:** she's so beautiful, so kind, simple…normal, in a word. I gave her a "French actress" look that I really like, a little jumbled, based all in navy blue… I also made up **Meryl Streep.** But the most beautiful woman I have ever worked on was **Brooke Shields:** she was 14 at the time and breathtaking. That skin, those lips, those eyes! That was my favorite photo shoot.

EXPRESS MAKEUP TIPS

AND SHE'S OFF! Five minutes before leaving the house… If you're blond with fair skin, don't go out without mascara. Similarly, a darker-skinned brunette cannot do without her lipstick. **My order:** **1:** hydrating base **2:** foundation **3:** blush **4:** eyeliner **5:** lips last: you can always touch up with a bit of gloss while stopping in front of a store window. **My secret weapon:** a small, all-in-one makeup kit, with five compartments: correcting cream, three shades of concealer, foundation, a bright blush for my cheeks, and my favorite lipstick. ▶

"Even in the evening, there's no need for exaggeration: I'm more about nuance than overstatement."

GOOD EVENING, MAKEUP KIT!

The difference between daytime and evening makeup is not as dramatic as you might think. Shinier lipstick and black rather than brown for the eyes usually suffice. Some women opt for more flashy, sparkly effects. I'm more about hints and nuances than overstatement.

BOBBI'S FAVORITE TRICKS

FOUNDATION There's only one reason to wear it: for a seamless complexion. To ensure that you have the right color, test a little on the side of your face, above your jaw. Depending on the occasion, you can choose a clear foundation or a bronzing powder. **EYEBROWS** should be in harmony with your face. If your facial features are pronounced, your brows should be too. If your face is more delicate, your eyebrow lines should be accordingly lighter. But they should always remain natural. Luckily we're no longer living in the age of brow massacres: waxed, plucked to death, or even shaved! **SUN** I'm one of the rare makeup artists to believe that sun brings out women's natural beauty. And protecting your skin (with maximum SPF facial sunscreen) never stopped anybody from getting a pretty tan. **BLUSH** What's the right color? The one that appears when you pinch your cheeks. **EYES** To look as natural as can be, mascara should be as dark as possible. I like it the way I created mine: black, very black, and rich. Most women put too much importance on eyeshadow. I believe it should come after eyebrows, eyeliner, and mascara: those three are the real key. You must buy shadow in just the right color, and it should require no extra work: it is very difficult to subdue a very dark eyeshadow. **LIPS** The ideal lipstick color is the one that complements the natural color of your lower lip: if it blends well there, you can be sure it works. You can go lighter or brighter, but I wouldn't recommend going darker: it can age you and doesn't look as good. **HOLD IT!** Mixing your makeup (eyeliner + powder, foundation + powder) multiplies durability tenfold. Remove any oily residue before doing your eyelids. Using two blushes will keep it looking fresh: use a natural shade and a slighter lighter one on top, and it will last at least half the day. Don't forget to reapply concealer in the middle of the day…

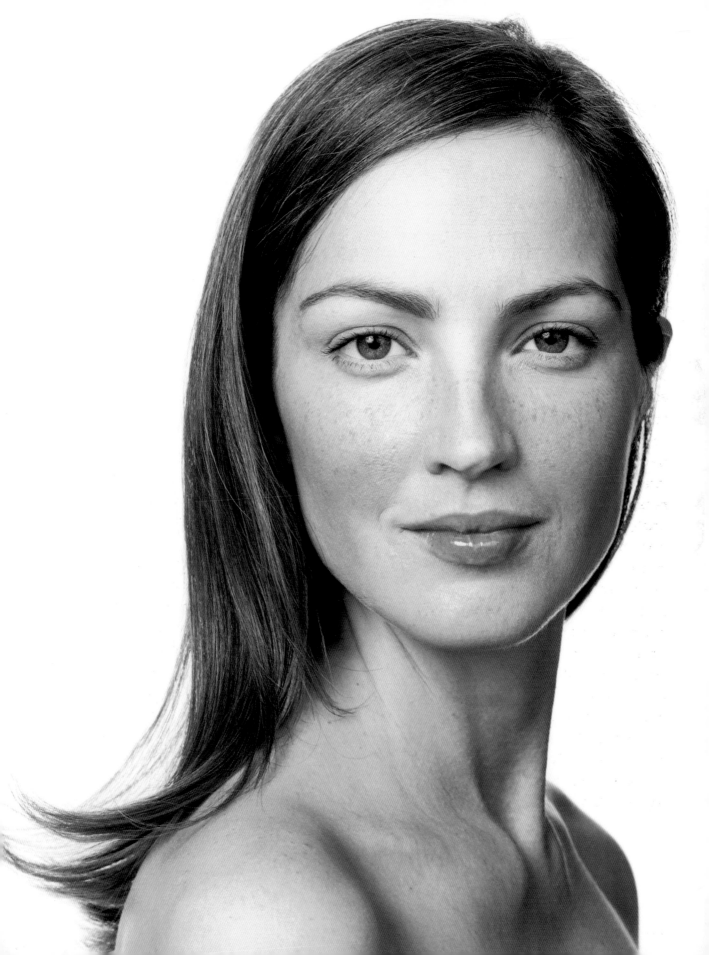

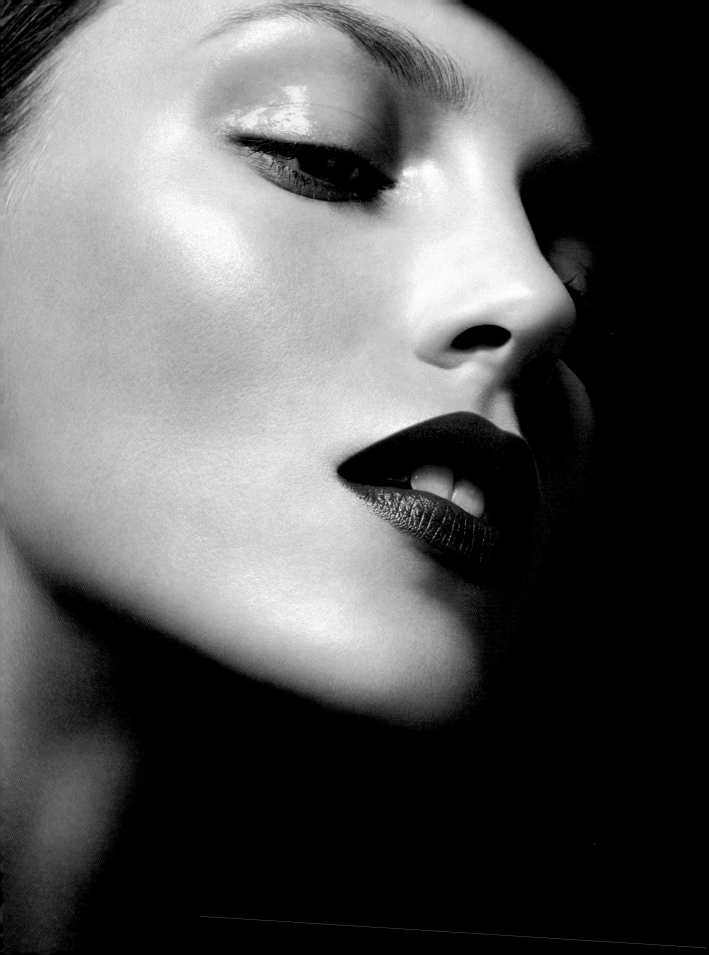

Giorgio Armani
Cosmetics

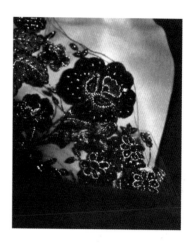

"Like fashion, makeup is an expression of femininity. It should be easy to apply yet still bring some element of fantasy." The Italian fashion designer goes from clothes to makeup with the same taste for airy materials and purity of color.

"There is nothing in the world more **sensual** than swathing a **body** in **fabric** and wrapping a **face** in a **veil** of smooth **textures**."

"Makeup according to Armani? It's a wardrobe for the face that you pick according to your mood. The Italian designer's entire philosophy is in that one sentence, in a spirit of luxury and freedom: **"To be elegant is not to be noticed. It is to be unforgettable..."** Where to start? Every woman has her own approach to beauty. She wants to "be beautiful," and that's more fundamental than just highlighting her eyes or lips. Clients' expectations from the cosmetics industry have greatly changed. They're looking for professional-quality tools and techniques, all with radiance and lightness that are available to them on a day-to-day basis. No masks or rigid effects; it's all about luminous textures and a "no makeup" illusion. The more made up you are, the more natural you should appear; but it's a very meticulous "natural." No disrespect intended to audaciousness, makeup "for show," theatricality, or Hollywood glamour. More than just makeup, Armani's products are an extension of his clothing: pure and airy textures that melt beautifully into the skin, available in an array of Mediterranean shades, soft monochromes, and subtle harmonies. Micro-Fil™, an exclusive technology inspired by layering techniques used in the textile industry, incorporates extremely fine and luminous raw materials that allow for translucent colors and ultra-smooth textures that can be endlessly superimposed. What Giorgio Armani hopes to offer women is a palette that "will allow them to express the myriad nuances of their emotions."

▶

THE ART OF A NATURALLY LUMINOUS COMPLEXION

Laurent Martin, Face Designer, Giorgio Armani Cosmetics

MAGNIFY

1. On perfectly clean and moisturized skin, use base to get a flawless complexion: apply a thin layer with your fingertips, spreading from the center of the face outward. With your hand cupped in a half-circle, work upward with light pressure along the contours of your face, the sides of your nose, and your jaw: your facial features will be perfectly blended. **2.** Brush techniques (see page 171). **3.** To hide redness and small imperfections, as well as bags, pimples, or other signs of fatigue, apply concealer to the outer and inner corners of your eye and around the edges of your nose. With the help of a highlighting brush, apply a small amount to problem areas, and dab lightly with your fingertips so that the texture blends perfectly with your foundation.

ILLUMINATE

4. As soon as you attract light to a particular spot on your face, you "reveal" it by adding volume through optical illusion. According to your mood, all combinations are possible: nuances revealed by luminizers are true gems. These products will create a radiant glow and highlight your most prominent facial features—cheeks, forehead, inner eye corners, upper cheekbones, and under the eyebrow arches. **5.** Loose powder envelops your face in a radiant veil and reduces shine. Apply the powder liberally with a brush on the center of your face for a discreet and naturally luminous glow. For a more sophisticated look, apply the powder to your whole face, neck, and shoulders.

SHAPE AND CURVE

6. Creating depth means creating shadows and redesigning the contours of your face. Depending on the look you want, use copper- or pink-toned luminizing liquids. Apply below your cheekbones to make them stand out, on your temples, along your jawline, and on the sides and tip of your nose to

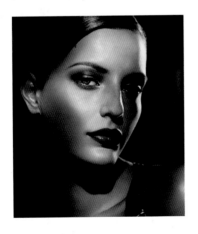

refine its volume. Use one dab of product for each zone and reapply as necessary. **7.** The final touch for a flawless complexion: sheer blush for a velvety finish or cream blush for a "no makeup" look. Apply in small dabs to your face, then blend with a brush. For instant freshness, apply in a figure-eight on your cheeks, or under your cheekbones for sophistication and glamour. Finally, bronzing powder can be swept on the center of your cheeks and the tip of your nose, the first places that natural sunlight would hit your face. ▶

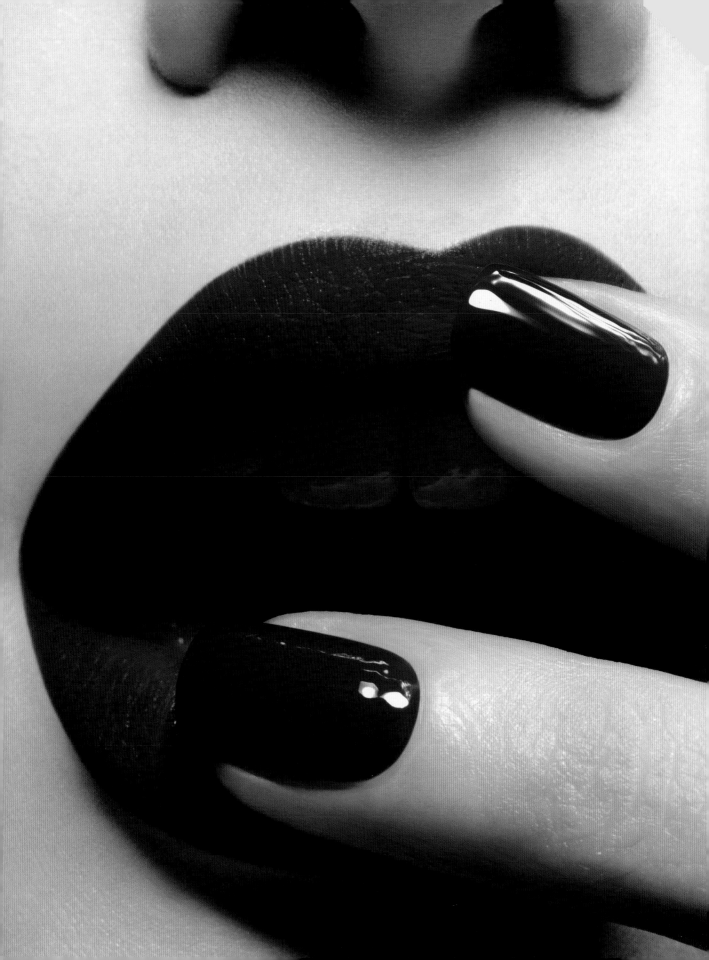

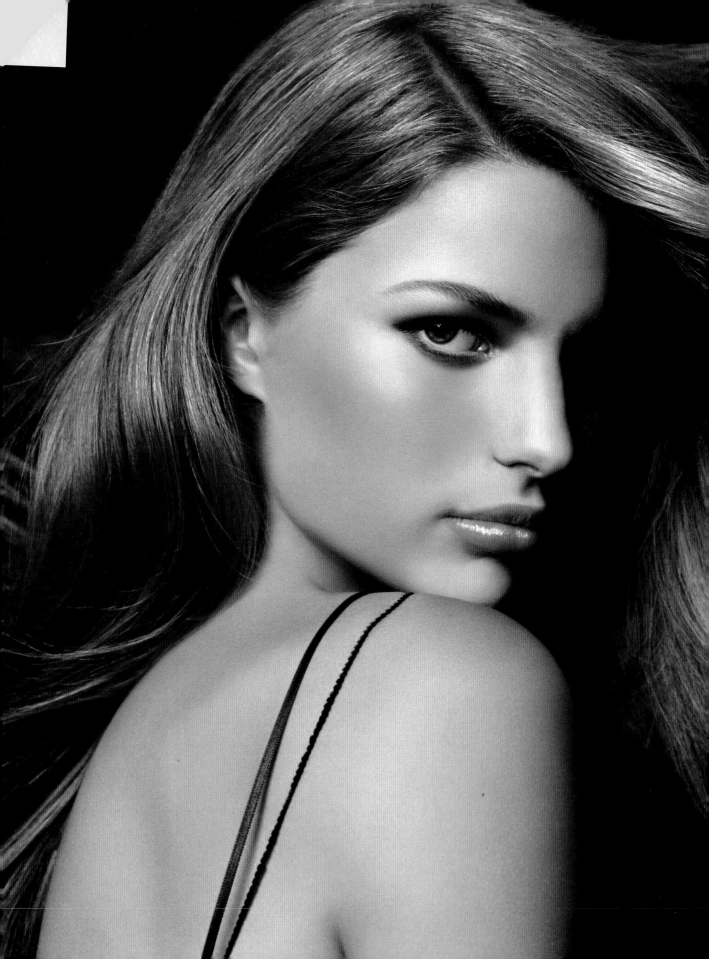

"My work consists not in superfluous add-ons but rather in purifying basics. Less is more."

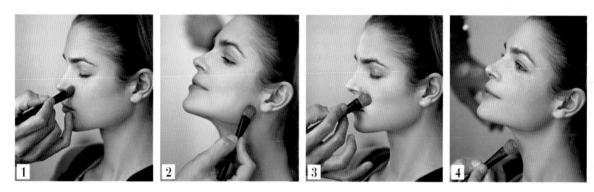

COMPLEXION: BRUSH TECHNIQUES. 1. Before applying foundation, warm the product up on the back of your hand with a foundation brush. Dot a small quantity of product on the tip of your brush. This technique allows you to control the intensity of your makeup according to the desired final look. Always start in the center of your face and work outward. **2.** Continue with broad strokes and spread the product outward with upward movements toward your hairline. **3.** Always work with a gentle foundation brush when dealing with sensitive spots where redness can develop, such as the sides of your nose, the outer corner of your eye, and the corners of your lips. **4.** Finish off with circular movements of the foundation brush from your jawline down to your neck.

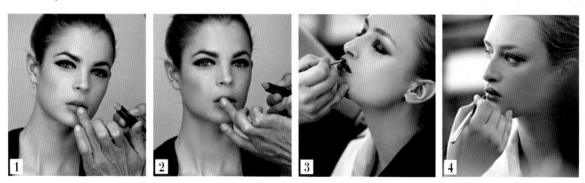

LIPS: NATURAL EFFECTS. 1. Prep your lips first with a sheer lipstick: opt for a transparent, shiny shade in beige or pink, and apply with your finger. **2.** End with your upper lip while tapping the middle of your lip for a "plumper" finish. **3.** For glamorous lips, prep them first with a sheer lipstick and redefine the contours of your lips with a smooth silk lip pencil for perfect lines. Blend the interior of your lips with a lip brush then apply a bold red, still using your lip brush. **4.** For an ultra-glamorous and sparkling finish, apply a glittery top coat to the middle of your lips. Sensual lips for a sophisticated finish… ▶

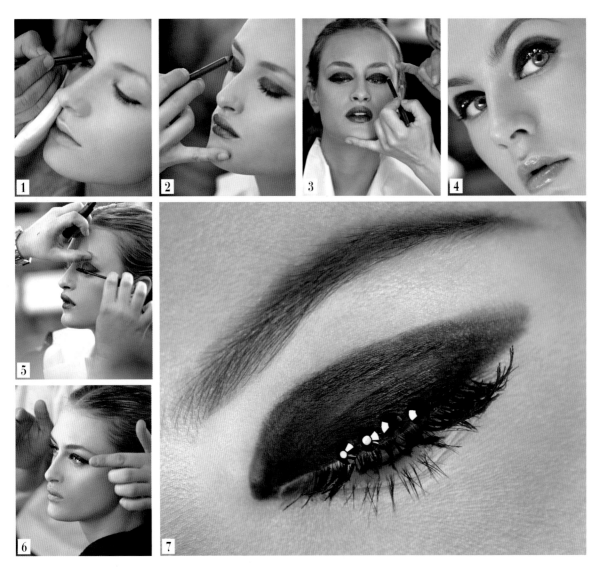

EYE GRAPHIC: BACKSTAGE IN MAKEUP. 1. Use a smooth silk eye pencil to sketch a line along your lashes. Define your workspace by drawing a line in the crease of your eyelid. **2.** Color in the entire eyelid up to the crease with the same pencil. For added sparkle, extend along to the outer corner of your eye. **3.** For greater depth, apply your eyeshadow as a fixer on top of the eyeliner. Use an eyeshadow brush and dot the product on lightly from the inside outward for a seamless finish. **4.** Using your silky smooth lip pencil, highlight the crease of your eyelid by extending color from the inner to the outer corner of your eye. With the help of an eye contour brush, use to-and-fro movements to blend the pencil. **5.** For a captivating gaze, use mascara with a curved brush, placing the curved end of the brush to the roots, covering the whole lash. Repeat, using the other end of the brush to add volume. **6.** To bring life to the corners of your eyes, set the makeup by tapping with the flat of your fingertip. **7.** Black crystals glued in the center of fake eyelashes are the ultimate final touch for sparkling sophistication.

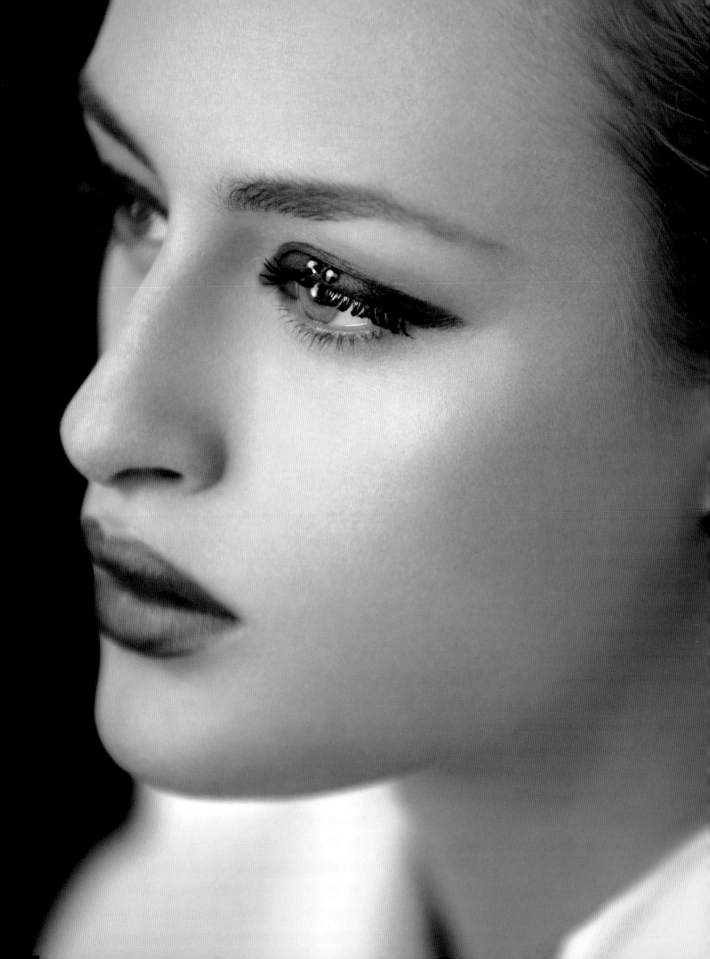

MAKEUP ARTISTS' SECRETS

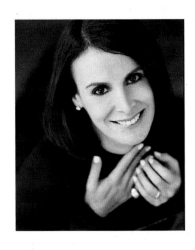

Terry
Founder of *by Terry*

A true star in the fashion industry, Terry's line is firmly established in the beauty market and has inspired the greatest haute couture designers. She opposes the standardization of the industry and stands for creativity and individuality.

"Makeup today is more about polishing your natural beauty than pseudo-perfection…"

What is modernity? A bare face with a few brilliant details, **lush lips,** spontaneous beauty… Getting it just right is the absolute key. Accentuate the light that is there naturally before trying to add more. I see no need for a foundation promising a supposedly flawless complexion. Today, women are using more and more makeup, and it shows less and less. No more masks: it's about showcasing what you've already got and using specific gestures to plump up, conceal, or **reveal your natural beauty.** In my opinion, makeup today is more about polishing your natural beauty than pseudo-perfection according to randomly defined rules of what's "beautiful." Everyone has natural beauty, and my philosophy is to respect and work with it. What I find interesting is when a woman who believes herself to be all too ordinary looks in the mirror and suddenly finds herself scintillating. Being attentive to women helps me to see that spark and make them feel less guilty. Every woman has a right—now, more than ever—to be a little narcissistic.   ▶

Terry's wildly rich palette showcased here, is like a cas full of dream-colored jewels

174

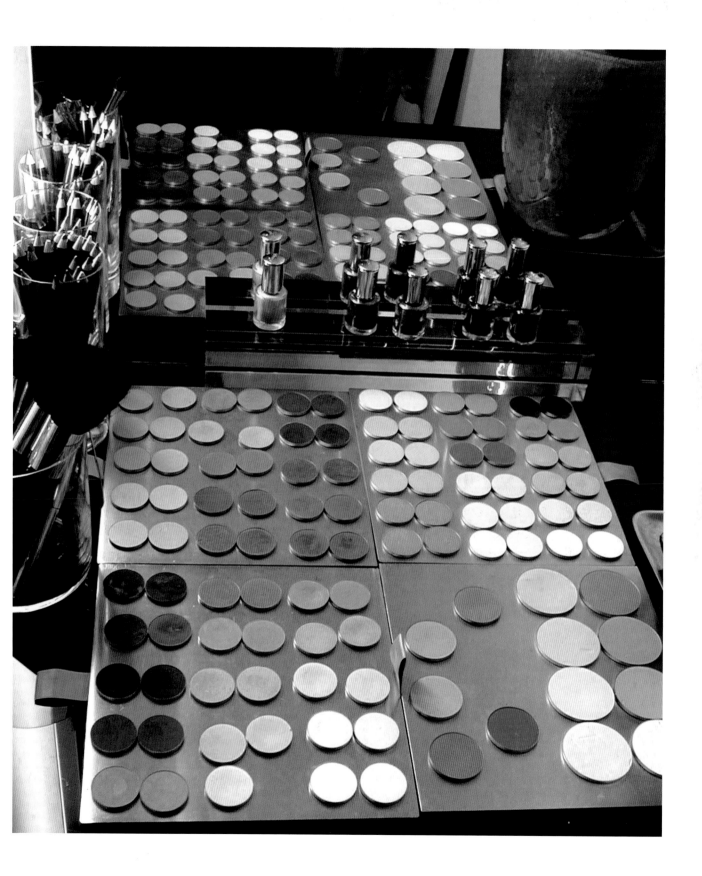

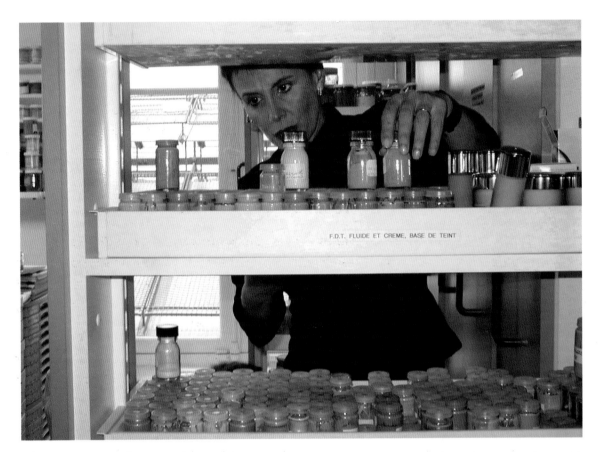

F.D.T. FLUIDE ET CREME, BASE DE TEINT

Terry in her secret laboratory.

You must feel good about yourself before trying to seduce others. No more stereotypes. The fashion industry has educated people: there are fewer catastrophes with beauty victims than with fashion victims! It's about controlled freedom, and you have to find your own way. You'll never be a professional, so don't try to become an at-home makeup artist. I'll give you a remote control with two buttons: "on" and "off." I'll deal with making it work. You just enjoy it!

INTERESTED IN A STUDIO SECRET?

I used to mix three products (foundation, hydrating cream, and smoothing gel) and place them around eyes and on necks: this gave immediate freshness to tired models. Using the Radiant touch (*Touche éclat*) brush that I designed at Yves St. Laurent in 1992, for example, delicately apply the mixture to your eye area, hollow of your chin, contour of your lips, and the sides of your nose.

"There are fewer catastrophes with beauty victims than with fashion victims"

TERRY'S TOUCH, LIVE FROM HER STUDIO

COMPLEXION My primary obsession is radiance! After the development of Color Skin Enhancer— veritable hours of sleep in a jar—my research team perfected a revolutionary formula enclosed in a gifted little brush called the Light-Expert Foundation Brush: it knows how to exfoliate! Its feather-light texture, eye-defying coverage, and innovative application make it the perfect foundation for every occasion. It comes in four zero-risk shades that suit virtually every skin tone.

Directions Click and dab the brush over areas needing light—under your eyes, on the tip of your chin, your cheekbones, forehead, and the sides of your nose. Blend with the brush and you have instant radiance. Try it: you can't go wrong!

CHEEKS A little pink on your cheeks is like a breath of fresh air. It raises your spirits and perks up your face. For a long time blush was controversial, but I have always believed in it and used it. It is freshness guaranteed and suits everyone: sublime on darker tones and delicate on fairer complexions.

EYES I like to set eyes against a dark backdrop much as a jeweller sets a precious stone. And mascara is a must! Generously cover the whole lash from root to tip. For the clumsy ones among you, I have a sure-fire tip for removing excess: dip a cotton swab in foundation. Roll and blend on the back of your hand. When used as a "corrector," it will dissolve mistakes without removing your makeup.

LIPS If your eye makeup is really pronounced, I would aim for more natural lips. If your eyes are more sober, then you can really shoot for the stars with your lips: plump them up with lip liner and blend with a brush.

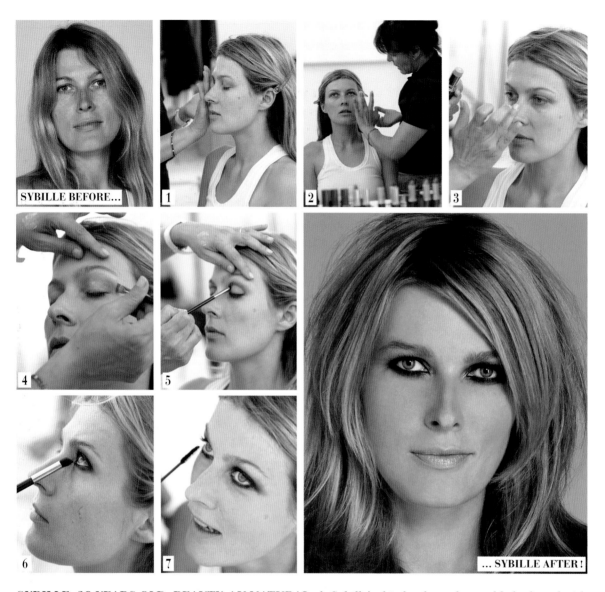

SYBILLE BEFORE...

1

2

3

4

5

6

7

... SYBILLE AFTER!

SYBILLE, 38 YEARS OLD, BEAUTY *AU NATURAL*. 1. Sybille's skin has been thoroughly hydrated with a rich cream. **2.** Since her face is lacking radiance, I generously applied a luminating liquid to create a play of light across her face. **3.** For a naturally flawless complexion, I used stick foundation on her prominent features and blended with my fingertips. This is an ideal way to hide all blemishes and imperfections. **4.** I've evened out her eyelids with mauve eyeshadow. **5.** With the help of a tapered brush, I've deepened her creases. **6.** I used the same color under her eyes. **7.** Her lower eyelashes are treated to a conditioning mascara to enlarge her eyes **...AND MADE OVER BY TERRY.** The contours of her face completely redefined, Sybille has reclaimed radiant skin. To attract attention to the rest of her face—and to avoid overdoing it—I've left her lips virtually untouched.

PATTY, 51 YEARS OLD, BEAUTY *AU NATURAL*. 1. and **2.** Patty's skin enjoys a long massage with cream. Her natural glow is already starting to emerge. **3.** Patty didn't want anything too heavy, so I applied fluid foundation with a brush. I top it off with loose powder. **4.** A pea-sized drop of liquid blush is applied transparently to the cheeks. **5.** Here I outline the eyes and then blend with a brush for a more natural look. I do the same work on the lower eyelids. **6.** Patty's eyelashes are covered in conditioning mascara. **7.** Finally, berry-toned lipcolor is dabbed on Patty's lips. **...AND MADE OVER BY TERRY.** Patty has been literally transformed. She has gained freshness and spontaneity. Her blue eyes stand out and her lips are unquestionably glamorous.

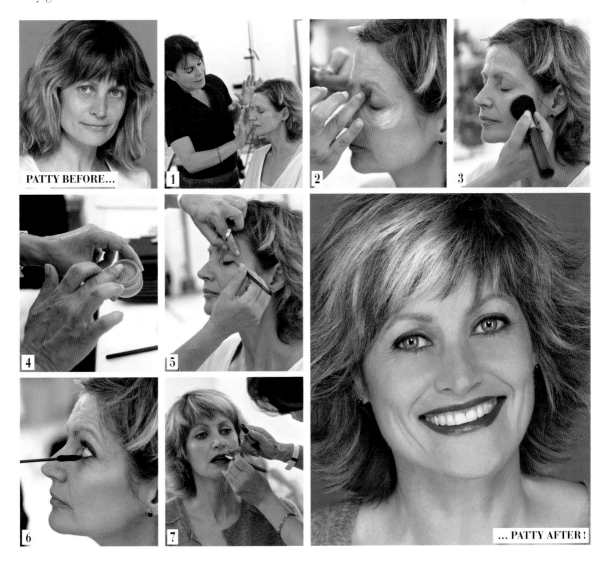

PATTY BEFORE...

1

2

3

4

5

6

7

... PATTY AFTER !

Night moves

7

BEAUTY AFTER DARK

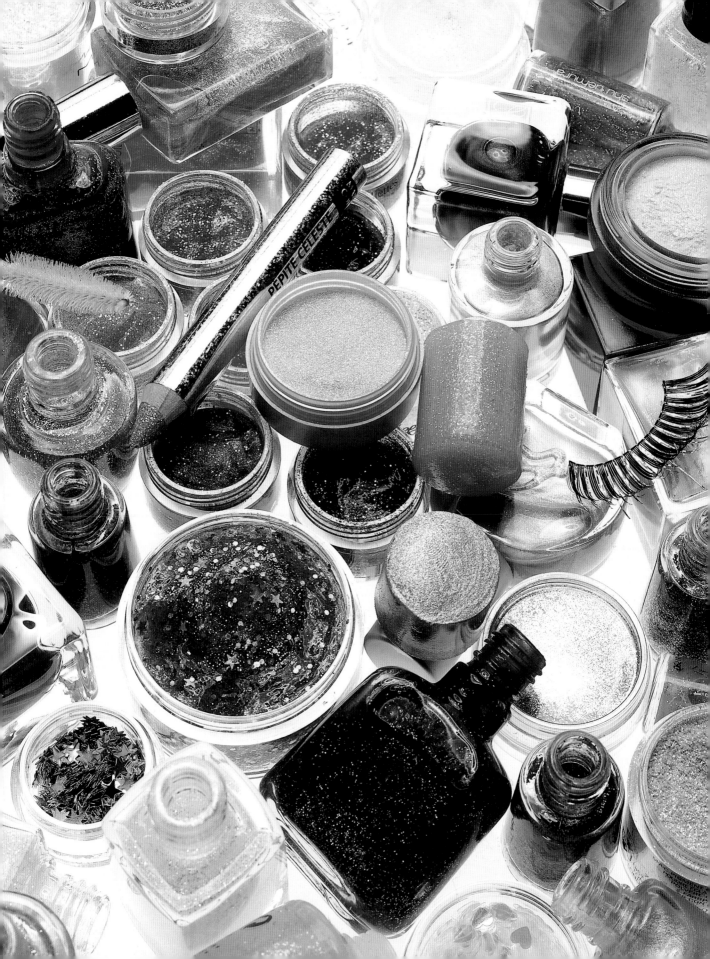

Stealthy panther or butterfly of the night— parties are meant for extremes.

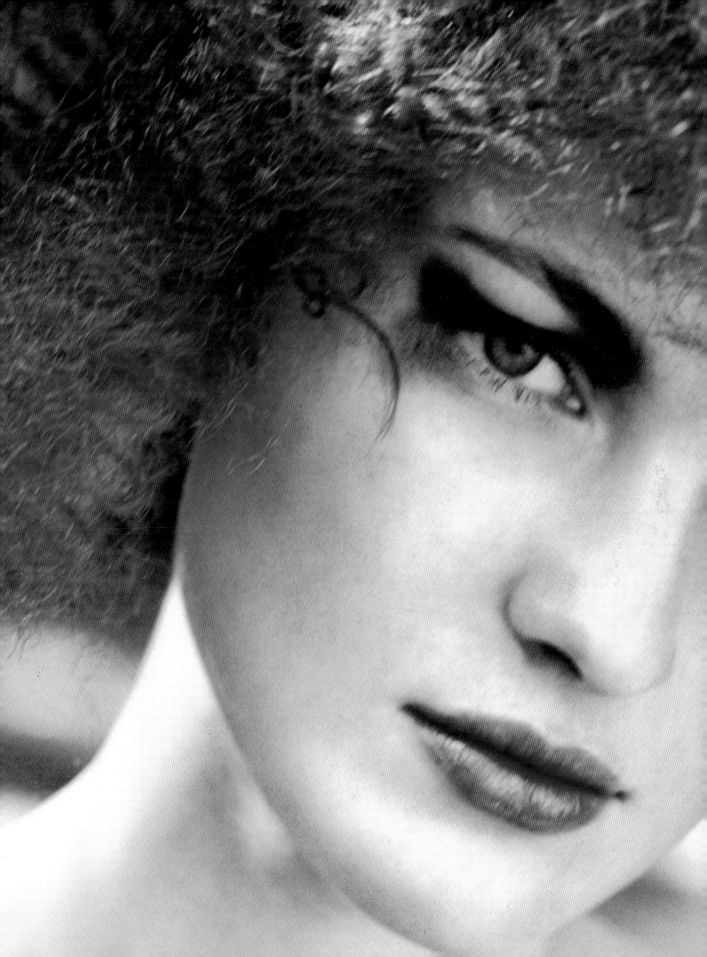

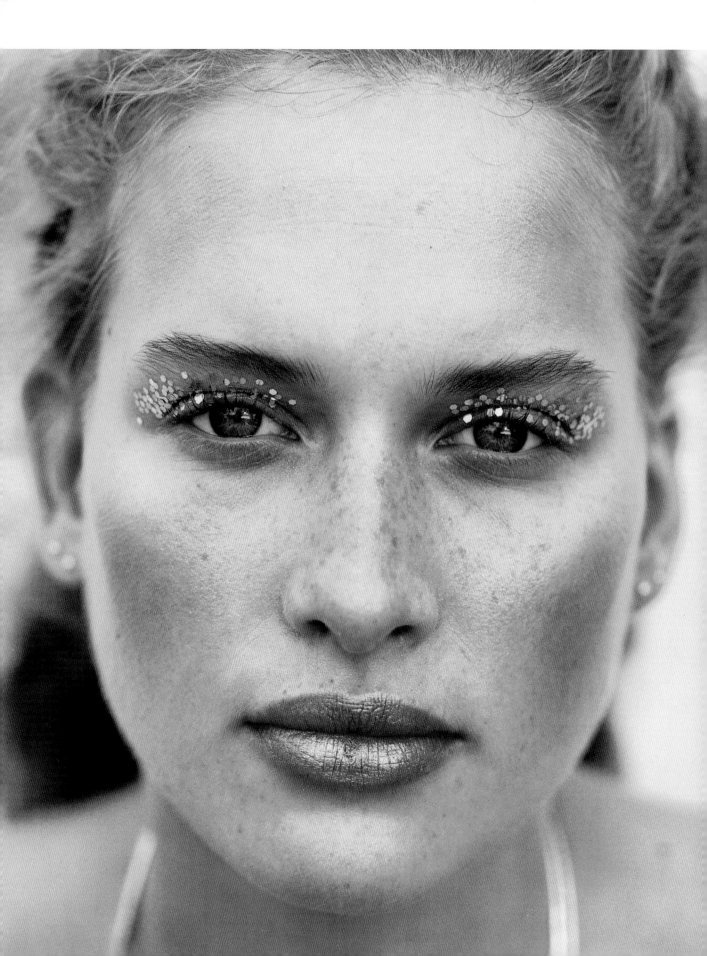

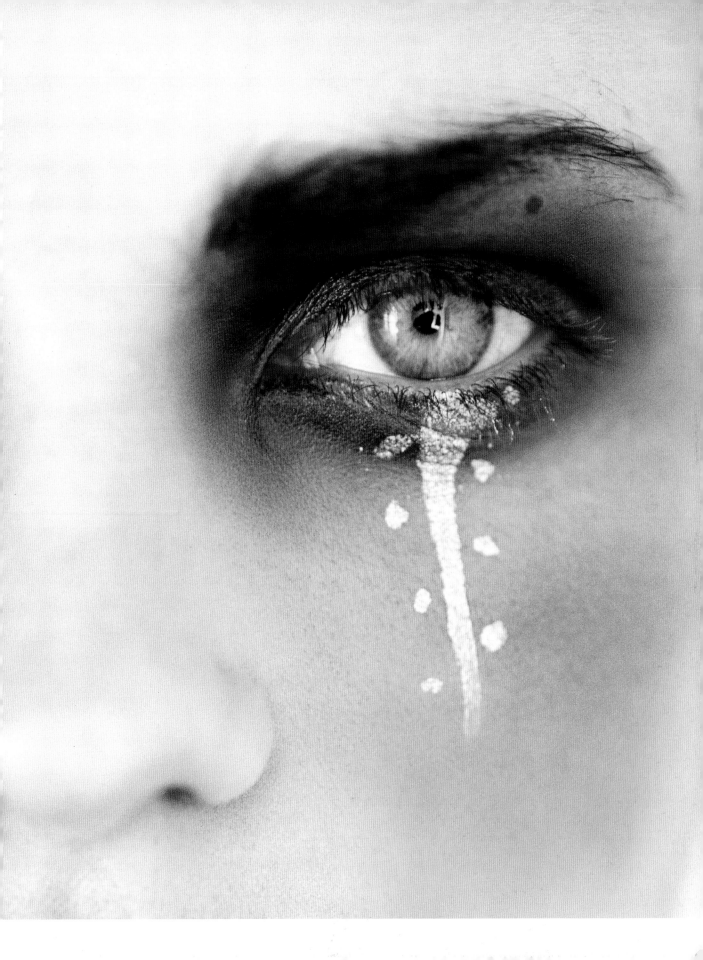

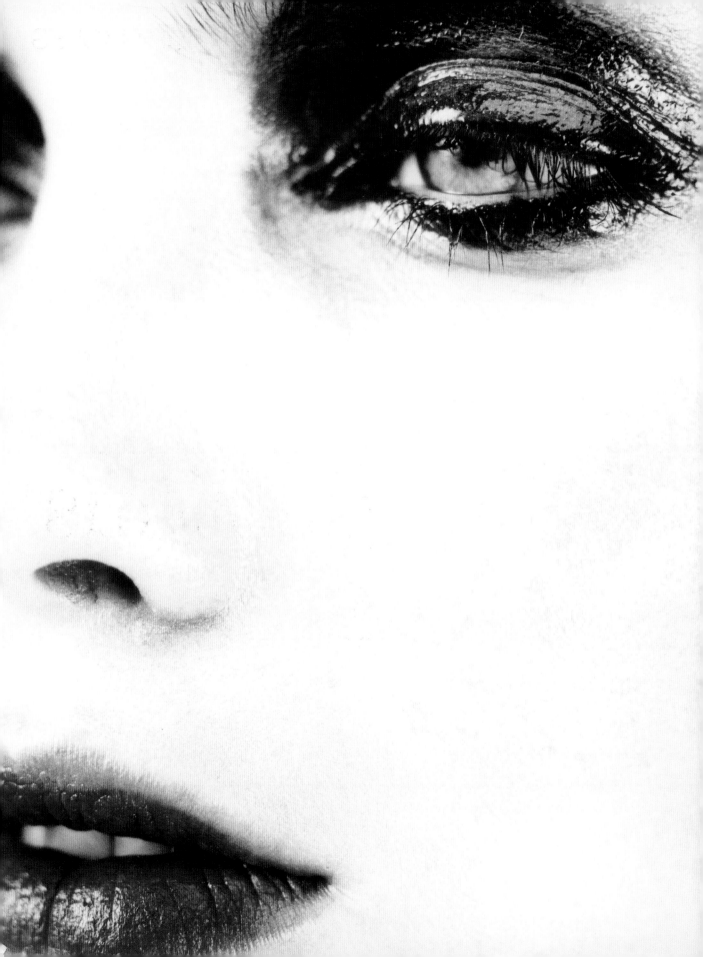

Deep —extreme— mysterious and chic

Special effects: Glitter and lights and everything nice

It's party time! Celebrate! Senses, colors, textures: offer your face intoxicating looks for that special night out.

GLITTER AND MAGICAL COLORS will make you gorgeous in the most unexpected of places. Shoulder-to-shoulder, above the strap of your heels, on your hairline, or above your cheekbone: don't be afraid to sparkle! Powder it on lightly after applying some essential oils—or on top of freshly-applied lip gloss.

LIQUID GOLD A simple streak of gold or silver eyeliner will change your look completely. Don't overdo it: you don't want to look like a Christmas tree! With a well-chosen colored mascara over a black kohl base on your lids, you'll instantly create a new look.

KOHL TATTOOS Who knew you were such a rebel…reserved for very special occasions.

What you'll need:
- essential body oil
- body paint
- glitter
- a whole lot of imagination!

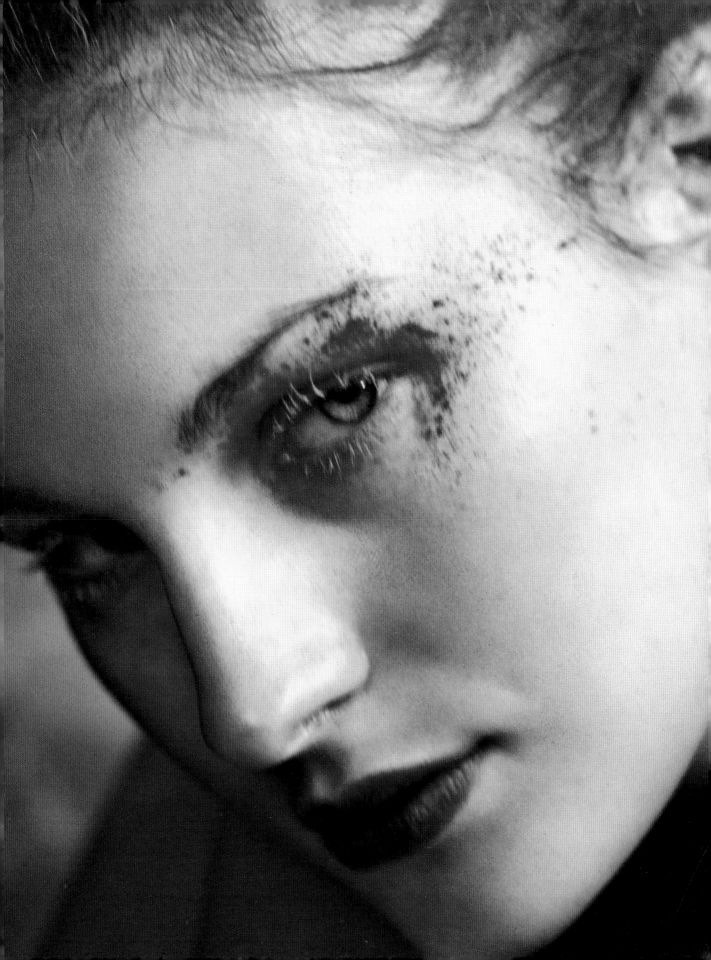

INDEX

PHOTO CREDITS

Cover: Front: Bruno Juminer. Back: Greg Conraux. Front Flap (left to right): Michael Wirth, Jeff Manzetti, Emmanuelle Hauguel; Back Flap (left to right): Sabine Villiard, Frédéric Farré, Jeff Manzetti. Hugh Arnold (p.66, 109). Aloïs Beer (p.34). Phil. Brazil (p.12b). Jean-Louis Colombel (p.64). Greg Conraux (p.44, 63, 95). Philippe Costes (p.124). Laurent Darmon (p.42, 126, 135). William Davies (p.58, 79). Thomas Dhellemmes (p.9, concept: Camille Soulayrol. creation: Johanna Elalouf). François Deconinck (p.38, 87, 92, 115). Essilor-Grrey (p.94a). Bruno Fabbri (p.82). Frédéric Farré (p.32, 48, 78, 90, 93, 96, 98, 100, 110, 122, 123, 129, 132, 137, 138, 139). Darren S. Feist/Marie Claire/IPC Syndication (p.71). Roberto Frankenberg (p.178, 179). Christian Giesen (p.16, 17, 18, 19, 20, 21). Hervé Haddad (p.12d). Emmanuelle Hauguel (p.35, 55, 67, 86, 86a, 104, 114, 119, 131, 184, 185). Frédéric Imbert (p.46, 47, 72, 88, 89). Bruno Juminer (p.40, 41, 120, 121). Eddy Kohli (p.183, 186, 189, 191). Wolfgang Ludes (p.12c, 31). Jeff Manzetti (p.12a, 26, 39, 43, 49, 52, 56, 76, 77, 91, 107, 130). Christopher Micaud (p.80). Marc Montezin (p.94b). Pascal Moraiz (p.24). Bob Norris (p.102, 117). Marc Philbert (p.23). Monika Robl (p.57, 84). Pierre Sabatier (p.181). Philippe Salomon (p.36, 37, 62, 65, 68, 70, 73, 74, 190). Michel Sedan (p.11a and b, 114). Jens Stuart (p.81). Liang Su (p.11c). Marcin Tyszka (p.29, 101). Sabine Villiard (p.45, 118, 136). Félix Von Muralt (p.140). Kenneth Willardt (p.11d, 30, 60, 112). Michael Wirth (p.85, 08). DR Guerlain (p.142–149). DR L'Oréal Paris (p.150–157). Gilles Traverso (p.153, 156a) Simon Procter (p.156.b and c, 157). DR Bobbi Brown (p.158–165). DR Giorgio Armani Cosmetics (p.166–173). DR By Terry (p.174–177).

MODEL CREDITS

Polly (p.115). Contrebande Patty (p.179). Élite Loan Chabanol (p.11b), Naomie Lan (p.45), Laura Cisneros (p.87, 117), Natalia Zavillova (p.183, 189, 191). Élite-Amsterdam Jolijn (p.26). First Model Anissa (p.63). Ford Jessica Van Der Steen (p.11d), Tessa Rolink (p.35), Micky Olin (p.40, 41, 120, 121). Idole Sarah Irvine (p.58). IMG Karin Anderson (p.12a, 43, 46, 47, 82), Svetlana Utkina (p.68, 70), Ana Muzica (p.77), Maria Lith (p.81, 110), Jacqueline Zao (p.85). Karin Zenia Eriksen (p.48), Kristina Semenovskaia (p.55), Lucie Novotny (p.122). Marilyn Katarina Scola (p.30), Sal Taylor (p.80). Metropolitan Fatou Ndiaye (p 11a, 114), Lu Yan (p.12d), Elena Soldatova (p.31), Laura Poketova (p.36, 37, 88), Danuta Nowowsiak (p.42), Olga Elnikova (p.65), Marina Prodnikava (p.108). Next Ilze Bajare (p.29, 101), Anja Rubik (p.60, 112), Nanda Hampe (p.109), Kelly Scott (p.184). Next-New York Caroline Eggert (p.49). Premier Model Management-Londres Yana Boyko (p.84). Woman Agnès Dhaussy (p.16, 18, 20, 21), Alyson (p.16, 19, 21). Women direct Arantxa Santa Maria (p.56, 76, 130), Alzbeta Syrovatkova (p.73, 190), Connie Houston (p.92), Marga Van Leen (p.135). Sybille Kleber (p.178).

Original title: Make Up
Copyright ©2006 by Éditions Marie Claire-Société
d'Information et de Créations (SIC)
www.marieclairebooks.com

General Director, Marie Claire Album SA:
   Arnaud de Contades
President, Marie Claire Album SA:
   Évelyne Prousost-Berry

Production Editor: Thierry Lamarre
Author and Editorial Director: Josette Milgram
English Translation: Christopher Bouchard with
   Melanie Molnar
Creative Director and Layout Designer: Valérie Paturel
Copy Editor: Julie Bavant
Editorial Assistant: Adeline Lobut
Art Department: Domitille Peyron, Sylvie Creusy,
   Isabelle Teboul

Library of Congress Cataloging-in-Publication Data
Marie Claire makeup / from the editors of Marie Claire
magazine.
     p. cm.
   Includes index.
   ISBN-13: 978-1-58816-668-5
   ISBN-10: 1-58816-668-6
   1. Cosmetics. 2. Beauty, Personal. I. Marie Claire
magazine.
   RA778.M329 2007
   646.7'2—dc22
                                        2007009283

10 9 8 7 6 5 4 3 2 1

Published by Hearst Books
A Division of Sterling Publishing Co., Inc.
387 Park Avenue South, New York, NY 10016

Marie Claire is a trademark of, and is used under license
from, Marie Claire Album. Hearst Books is a trademark
owned by Hearst Communications, Inc.

www.marieclaire.com

Distributed in Canada by Sterling Publishing
c/o Canadian Manda Group, 165 Dufferin Street
Toronto, Ontario, Canada M6K 3H6

For information about custom editions, special sales,
premium and corporate purchases, please contact Sterling
Special Sales Department at 800-805-5489 or
specialsales@sterlingpub.com.

Manufactured in China

Sterling ISBN 13: 978-1-58816-668-5
        ISBN 10: 1-58816-668-6